Graduate Professional Education Through Outreach: A Nursing Case Study

Graduate Professional Education Through Outreach: A Nursing Case Study

DOROTHY E. REILLY

Pub. No. 15-2340

National League for Nursing

This book was set in Astor by Publications Development Company. The editor and designer was Allan Graubard. Clarkwood Corporation was the printer and binder.

The cover was designed by Lillian Welsh.

Printed in the United States of America

Contents

About the Author

Preface

1 Professional Education Through Outreach Programs:
   Examining the Concept   1

2 Developing a Quality Outreach Program:
   Assessing the Feasibility   9

3 Design of a Quality Outreach Program:
   The Community-Based Model   23

4 Strategies for Organization and Administration   43

5 Faculty: An Important Key to Quality   59

6 Strategies for Delivery of an Outreach Program   73

7 Teaching Skills Specific to Graduate Professional Education:
   Specialized Clinical Practice and Research   97

8 Issues in Budgeting an Outreach Program   109

9 Outcomes: What Was the Impact of the Outreach Program
   on the Graduates?   133

10 Outcomes: What Was the Impact of the Outreach Program
   in the Communities Involved?   155

References   173

Appendix A. Questionnaire for Alumnae   177

Appendix B. Clinical Course Evaluation Survey   189

Appendix C. Research Skills Questionnaire   193

About the Author

Dorothy E. Reilly, EdD, RN, FAAN, has been a significant force in nursing education for many years. She has taught at Boston University School of Nursing, Columbia University School of Nursing, and is currently Professor Emeritus at Wayne State University, College of Nursing. She is a noted author in the field of nursing education with numerous books and articles to her credit.

For almost 12 years Dorothy E. Reilly held the post of Director of Outreach Programs at Wayne State University, an experience foundational to the breadth of this book. She has also been a consultant to other Colleges of Nursing that offer outreach programs at the baccalaureate and graduate level.

Preface

Although equal access to higher education is valued in our society, impediments to its achievement still exist. Whether these impediments result from structural, philosophical, economic, or educational concerns, their general effect is similar. Geography also must be considered in this list. This case study report concerns the impediment of geography. It discusses the approaches which one institution of higher learning, Wayne State University, used in meeting the higher educational needs for a specific population of health profession students in five selected sites in the state of Michigan.

Geography is a relational factor. Obviously, there exists a relationship between the location of an institution of higher learning and the population requiring access to the programs offered. The higher the educational level, the more serious becomes the issue of accessibility. Community college education, for example, is relatively accessible throughout the state. Institutions offering a baccalaureate program are generally more limited but available to many communities. The presence of a baccalaureate degree granting institution does not necessarily mean that programs needed by a community will be offered, however. This is of special concern when professional or other highly specialized programs are needed in communities.

It is at the graduate level that the impediment of geography becomes a grave concern. Because of the nature of graduate study and the resources required, the number of institutions providing such programs is limited. Although many communities need the knowledge and expertise which constitute these programs, many of their constituencies are limited in the mobility required to attend such programs on campus. Graduate preparation in the professions, especially in fields of health and human resources, is essential to meet needs of communities, yet such programs are the least likely to be available beyond selected campus areas.

Resolution of the geographical access problem could involve the development of more graduate programs so as to increase availability to a larger

The outreach program was partially supported by advanced training grants, #2D23 NU 00245, Division of Nursing, Health Resources and Services Administration, Department of Health and Human Services, Public Health Service.

constituency. Such an approach, except on a broad basis, may be question-able since there is a finite dimension to the availability of resources such programs would require. Another approach involves the delivery of quality graduate programs into selected regions by the established institutions of higher learning.

It is the latter approach that the College of Nursing, Wayne State University, used to meet critical demands of outstate regions in Michigan for graduate prepared teachers, administrators, clinical practitioners, and researchers in nursing so as to serve the health needs of their population.

A community-based model which depicts a reciprocal relationship between Wayne State University and the communities involved was developed and served as an operative and decision-making framework in five different regions in the state. Although developed for a specific professional program, the model is appropriate for use in any outreach effort regardless of the program.

This report presents the philosophical, programmatic, procedural, financial, and organizational concerns as Wayne State University engaged in this outreach endeavor. Data from extensive evaluation protocols for the first four programs and a comprehensive questionnaire responded to by 79 percent (154/196) graduates are incorporated throughout the text. The fifth outreach program was not completed at this writing.

Chapter 1 presents various concepts about outreach programs and the special demands of professional education.

Chapter 2 examines the issue of providing a quality outreach program in terms of community need, factors involved in identifying an available pool of students, demographic area of a student, and other matters which influence programmatic decisions. Questions of the meaning of commitment on the part of the sponsoring institution from a moral perspective are raised.

Chapter 3 introduces several models of outreach programs as they reflect the beliefs and operational practices of sponsoring institutions. The community-based model used by the College of Nursing, Wayne State University, is presented and its implementation in the various sites is described in terms of criteria of the model and issues raised.

Chapter 4 presents elements in designing an administrative framework for implementing outreach programs which integrate on-campus and on-site processes. The use of the administrative framework developed by the College of Nursing is presented and some of the problems which arose are discussed.

Chapter 5 addresses the issues relating to faculty appointment in off-campus teaching in terms of qualifications, and processes and procedures to assure that the quality of teaching personnel is the same for students in both on-campus and off-campus programs. The practices used in the community-based model are described and evaluated from student, graduate, and faculty perspective.

Chapter 6 examines strategies in the delivery of graduate professional outreach programs from the perspective of governing policies, procedures, and modifications as indicated. The scheduling patterns used by the College of Nursing in the outreach program and issues related to content and method-ologies of teaching are presented. Faculty, student, and graduate evaluations of the various elements in the delivery of the program are included.

Chapter 7 addresses the teaching of the two skills specific to graduate professional education, specialized clinical practice and research. Strategies and processes used and the faculty, student, and graduate evaluations of their experiences constitute the substance of the chapter.

Chapter 8 identifies issues in budgeting an outreach program and pre-sents an analysis of cost factors as they relate to the budget processes in the sponsoring institution. Cost items unique to outreach programs are discussed in terms of the outreach model used by the institution.

Chapter 9, using data primarily from the graduate questionnaire, devel-ops a professional profile of the graduates. Findings on all professional behavior variables used denote that an outreach program can provide for professional socialization of its students.

Chapter 10, using multiple data sources, identifies the impact that the outreach program has had on the communities where it was located and on the College of Nursing and Wayne State University.

Finally this book is written in acknowledgement of the commitment and efforts of those people who enabled the College of Nursing to demonstrate that a quality graduate professional outreach program can address inequities in the geographical distribution of professionals so as to meet particular service needs within communities. Students and faculty united and preserved in their belief that a quality educational experience could be a reality even though a program was offered in regions far removed from the main campus. Families of students also deserve recognition for their role in supporting the students and the program in spite of the temporary disruption in their lifestyles. Special recognition goes to all those persons and agencies in the various outreach sites who made the notion of a community-based program model a dynamic phe-nomenon. The continued support and guidance from the Dean of the College of Nursing in concert with members of the administrative staffs of the college and university enabled the program to proceed with integrity and adherence to the standards of these institutions.

All participants are particularly grateful to the staff in the Division of Nursing, Health Resources and Services Administration, Department of Health and Human Services, United States Public Health Service for their continued belief in this endeavor, advice, and financial support without which this pro-gram could not have come to fruition.

Special individuals have made significant contributions to this manu-script. Thomas Templin, research assistant in the Center for Health Research, College of Nursing, assisted with the preparation of the alumnae questionnaire and the statistical management of the data. The author is particularly indebted to three persons who served as continuous expert viewers and critics of the manuscript, contributing to the clarity of the presentation, the quality of the content, and the total effect of the manuscript. These three professionals are:

Lorene Fischer, Dean of the College of Nursing, Wayne State University, Maria Phaneuf, Professor emeritus, College of Nursing, Wayne State University, and Dr. Patricia Moritz, Nurse Consultant, Advanced Training Programs, Division of Nursing Bureau, Health Resources and Services Administration, Department of Health and Human Services who is now Chief of the Nursing Systems Branch, National Center for Nursing Research.

The College of Nursing, Wayne State University, took a risk when it offered its graduate professional program through outreach. It is a pleasure to share the success of this experience with colleagues and others interested in using this approach in addressing inequities in the geographic distribution of professionals wherever and in whatever discipline this phenomenon occurs.

Dorothy E. Reilly, EdD, RN, FAAN
Director of the Outreach Program

1

Professional Education
Through Outreach Programs:
Examining the Concept

To alleviate nursing shortages in medically underserved areas, their residents need better access to all types of nursing education, including outreach and off-campus programs. (p. 164)

The above quotation is one of the conclusions of the 1983 report of the Institute of Medicine, *Nursing and Nursing Education: Public Policies and Private Actions.* Although nursing is identified, there are many other health professions to which such a statement might apply—in most of these professions, maldistribution of their practitioners and resources is an ongoing phenomenon. Clustering of expertise occurs around the larger metropolitan areas, leaving the roughly 30 percent of the population dwelling in rural and semirural areas with sparse professional services often provided by inadequately prepared individuals.

The conclusion stated in the above report not only includes the finding, *nursing shortages in medically underserved areas,* it also proposes action: *provide better access to all types of nursing education, including outreach and off-campus programs.* The implications of such a recommendation are many, and they need to be explored by those contemplating action in the proposed direction.

1

CONCEPT OF OUTREACH PROGRAM

Programs offered away from the main campus of an institution of higher learning are referred to by such titles as : *external degree, off-campus, satellite, outreach.* The term, *external degree,* connotes a state that does not exist in reality. Although the program leading to the degree may occur external to the main campus, the degree itself remains constant in the degree granting institution. A precise definition of the term does not exist, but it generally implies a nontraditional approach to education which is offered off-campus to an adult population. Cross (1973) identifies the central elements to the concept: "Learning is defined as quality of student rather than the offerings of the college. Interest is greater in what has been learned than in what has been taught. Education is student centered" (p. 48).

Bowen (1973) refers to the external degree as a "degree granted by a college or university, or other institutions on the basis of learning acquired partly, mainly or wholly outside the degree granting institutions" (p. 480). A more narrow view of the term, *external degree,* is expressed by Warren (1973) as he proposes ways to award credit for previous experiences. His approach suggests a degree awarded for competencies developed independently of the degree granting institution, such as occurs in the New York Regents External Degree Program.

The more usual pattern of external program involves a closer relationship between the off-campus and on-campus programs where courses and standards are the same, but differences may occur in methodologies and scheduling patterns. A more precise definition of the various types of external programs may be stated, however. The term, *off-campus,* offers only a limited perspective, for it suggests primarily a geographic connotation; programs may be in any location not identified as part of the main campus. The term, *satellite,* refers to a program in a setting away from the main campus where the overall operations are administered by the parent organization. The term, *outreach,* however, is a dynamic concept based on the definition of Webster, "the act of reaching out." Since the word, *campus,* is not included in this concept, a different definition of campus may be noted; a community or geographical area with all of its varied resources can be perceived as the campus for a particular program.

The term, *external program,* is an appropriate one and encompasses the other terms, *off-campus, satellite,* and *outreach.* The University of Michigan conducted a feasibility study (Eisley & Coppard, 1977) regarding external graduate degree programs using the definition, "External graduate programs are graduate programs characterized by methods of instruction and organization that make them available to students constrained from attending traditional residential programs" (p. 8).

Another dimension in categorizing the type of external program to be offered is the degree of permanency of the program in a specific area. Often an off-campus program designates a degree of permanency where courses are offered on an ongoing basis as long as the enrollment of students justifies its existence. A satellite program represents a relatively permanent status since it is a setting managed, staffed, and controlled by the parent institution. Since an outreach program generally does not have a designated base in a community, it is often considered as a temporary program where access is for a designated period of time.

The intent of the sponsoring agency in offering a program away from its main campus will define the meaning and purpose. The outreach concept seems compatible with the intent stated in the 1983 Institute of Medicine report for it addresses the educational access issue in regions where none presently exist and where practitioner mobility to attend campus programs is restricted. Upgrading of professional preparation in a community through outreach programs often enables the community to develop at a later date its own programs. The term used primarily in this presentation is *outreach*.

PROFESSIONAL EDUCATION

Education of the health professional is the prerogative of the college or university and entails both a theoretical and practice domain. While professional education in the health professions is specialized, it also incorporates the knowledges and skills reflective of the general liberal arts education. However, a deliberate socialization directed toward the role behaviors and values of the particular profession is involved. It requires the development of cognitive, psychomotor, and affective skills inherent in practice to a level of professional competency and, in graduate education, the development of research capability.

Professionals practice under a social mandate: their services are viewed as beneficial to society. This mandate means that professional activities are subject to scrutiny by the society and all professionals are accountable to practice in accord with the values, standards, and expectations of society. Thus, a professional program must be concerned not only with the development of specialized expertise inherent in the practice, but also with the development of the total person who must interact with various individuals and political and social groups within the larger society.

Schlotfeldt (1987) describes the significant criterion for identifying professionals: "those who so qualify have mastered and are able to use in practice judiciously, skillfully, humanly, and ethically, an agreed upon body of knowledge that is fundamental to the fulfillment of nursing's social mission" (p. 228). Although nursing was the referent here, the criterion applies to any profession.

Professional education may occur in baccalaureate, master's, and doctoral programs in accord with accepted practices of the particular profession. The first professional degree usually prepares the generalist while advanced degrees prepare the specialist and researcher.

In nursing, the baccalaureate degree program is usually the preparation for entering the profession as a generalist and is often referred to as a generic program. Two types of students enter this program: (1) those embarking on a nursing career and (2) those who are already licensed to practice as registered nurses but are returning to school as they change their career goals from technical practice (associate or diploma preparation) to professional practice (baccalaureate preparation). It is for this latter group of students that an outreach baccalaureate program is likely to be offered. Each school offering such a baccalaureate program has a procedure by which advanced standing may be allocated for previous experiences; so that the program must be flexible enough to meet individual needs of students since all will not be at the same point in the program when they enter.

Graduate study in nursing is generally geared to the preparation of specialists (there are a few graduate programs that prepare for entry into the profession at the graduate level). This preparation is directed toward the skills of advanced practice which is characterized by Diers (1985) as "depth over breath and specific over general" (p. 43). Diers sees decision making as the critical behavior in advanced practice, which is dependent upon three kinds of knowledge: clinical judgment, scholarly inquiry, and leadership. It is to graduates from such programs that the profession looks for leadership for change since their acceptance by society as experts places them in a fortuitous position to influence policies and practices within the community.

Two aspects of graduate professional education are implied: (1) the need for a practice component to develop the requisite competencies of an expert and (2) research experience to contribute as generators and implementers of new nursing knowledge as it evolves. Reilly (1985) states, "The charge to educators of professionals is to prepare practitioners who not only possess the requisite knowledge and skills inherent in their practice, but who also have the ability to evolve their own theory of practice which is congruent with the expectations of the discipline as it interfaces with society."

It is the particular nature of professional education that causes some faculties to question the feasibility of offering such a program in an outreach site. Questions such as the following arise: Can the quality of the program be maintained when removed from the resources of the institution and the usual health care agencies in the area? How can professional socialization occur when students are not interacting with faculty and students on a regular basis? How can such a program be delivered, monitored, and result in the same product as the on-campus programs? Will the clinical practice experiences be of comparable quality to those provided on campus? In essence, can a quality professional education program be offered as an outreach program? It is the intent of this presentation to demonstrate that an affirmative response to the questions is possible.

PROGRAMS VS. COURSES IN OUTREACH

The word, *program*, rather than courses is used thus far to emphasize those deliberatively planned educational experiences which in their totality lead to the attainment of a degree. The offering of selected courses in a region may contribute to the continuing education needs of a population, but it is the ability to meet degree requirements that is most needed by professionals in outreach sites. Continuing education is necessary for upgrading ongoing practice of professionals and may be obtained in a community by various means other than courses. The availability of courses is of less concern. It is the availability and accessibility of a quality professional program leading to a degree, undergraduate or graduate, that is addressed here. Issues to be raised by individuals contemplating such an effort are philosophical, theoretical, and pragmatic.

OUTREACH PROGRAM:
COLLEGE OF NURSING, WAYNE STATE UNIVERSITY

Twelve years of experience of the College of Nursing, Wayne State University, in offering a Master of Science in Nursing Outreach Program in five different locations in Michigan have provided much data pertinent to the issue concerned with taking graduate professional degree programs to sites removed from the campus. The design of the college's program was based on the concept of mass preparation of professionals in a community. A program was brought to an outreach site for a one-time event where a large number of people were prepared at the same time during a two- or three-year period. At the conclusion of the designated time period, the college moved the program to another site. A total of five different sites in Michigan have been involved in this endeavor (see Table 1 & Figure 1).

Data obtained from the total experience comprise a critical component of this report. An extensive questionnaire to assess the graduates' perspective of the impact of the outreach program on themselves and the community was sent to 195 graduates during January and February, 1986. Two graduates from the program are deceased. Following the initial mailing, a second mailing was sent to the nonrespondents. A third follow up comprised a letter sent to the individuals who had not answered the first two

Table 1
Outreach Program Sites

Date	Location	Miles from Campus	No. of Students
6/1/75–12/31/77	Upper Peninsula Michigan	486	35
1/1/77–12/31/79	Western Michigan	157	58
1/1/80–12/31/81	HSA VI (Mid-Eastern Michigan)	103	63
3/1/82–2/28/85	HSA VII (Upper Western Michigan)	256	39
3/1/85–2/28/87	*HSA III (South West Michigan)	145	68
Total			263

*In process

Figure 1
Location of Outreach Programs

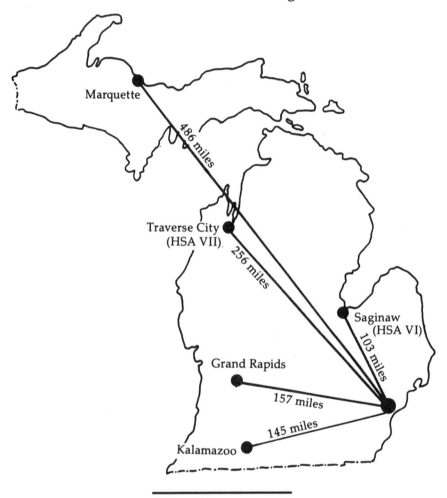

requests. The data pool used in this report is 154 responses or 79 percent from graduates. It is recognized that on some questions there may be some variability in the number of responses.

The allocation of responses according to the location of the program is noted in Table 2.

When relevant, data from the 68 students currently in the fifth program are used and so identified.

Table 2
Number of Respondents per Program to Questionnaire

Location	No. of Respondents	% of the Group
Upper Peninsula	27	75
Western Michigan	51	88
Tri-City (HSA VI)	44	70
Northwestern Michigan (HSA VII)	32	82
Total	154	

CONCLUSION

Access to educational programs which lead to a degree is often a geographical problem which results in maldistribution of prepared professionals throughout many regions of our society.

Several mechanisms have been developed which enable degree granting institutions to bring programs to underserved areas. These programs appear under various titles such as external degree, off-campus, satellite, and outreach.

Professional educational programs, whether at the baccalaureate or graduate level, have unique elements which lead some individuals to decide that they can be offered only within the resources of the on-campus environment. The need to prepare persons with specialized competencies that are practiced under a social mandate to provide service to communities requires that a practice component be an integral part of the total program. At the graduate level of professional education the program must provide for not only the development of specialized expertise, but also, research skills. This fact is often perceived as a deterrent to offering graduate professional programs in outreach locations.

The College of Nursing, Wayne State University, has offered a Master of Science in Nursing program in five different underserved areas in Michigan. Data from this experience including responses from 154 of the 195 living graduates to an extensive questionnaire are used in response to the question: Can a quality graduate professional program be offered on off-campus sites? What follows is a case study of an outreach effort with graduate programs in a health care profession.

2

Developing a Quality Outreach Program: Assessing the Feasibility

Should a school or college offer an outreach program? Each individual institution of higher learning must make the decision on the basis of demonstrated need in the designated areas and the commitment to this endeavor that the institution is willing to affirm. This decision is not to be taken lightly if a program, comparable to the one on campus, is to be offered to residents in an outreach site. The commitment is also a moral one, for the institution must assure that individuals who enter the program will have the opportunity to complete requirements and be awarded the appropriate degree. Outreach programs are effective in increasing enrollment of students, a significant concern to many educational institutions during the 1980s and 1990s, but this factor cannot be the overriding determinant in embarking on this venture; for the institution must be prepared to assure that it has the resources to provide a quality program in the outreach site.

MEANING OF A QUALITY PROGRAM

What is a quality program? Is it possible to deliver a quality professional program in locations removed, often far removed, from the resources and academic climate of the main campus? This latter question has been posed by many educators and agencies responsible for monitoring the quality of educational programs.

External programs will not meet quality standards unless quality controls are built into the program design. The term, *quality program,* as it is used in outreach programs, derives its expression from the philosophy, goals, and objectives of the sponsoring institution, for it is in this institution that the notion of quality is conceptualized and the process is monitored and controlled. Quality is related to the on-campus program; the standards and criteria by which it meets the requisites established by the sponsoring institution and accrediting bodies to which it is accountable. Quality means the *same* program is offered in the outreach site as approved for on campus.

The notion of *sameness* requires clarification, however, for it is often confused with the notion of *identical. Sameness* means that both programs are guided by the same objectives, have the same requirements, evaluative criteria, and are taught by faculty who fulfill the same appointment criteria. Control of the planning, development, and implementation of each program rests with the same groups within the institution's organization. Within this notion of sameness there is opportunity for flexibility so as to meet the specific needs of students and faculty involved in the outreach site. This flexibility may be in terms of patterns of class and course scheduling, organization of content and experiences to accommodate these different patterns, and the selection of experiences which maximize the resources of the community. Objectives are the constant variable, routes by which these objectives are attained may be altered in terms of the characteristics of the learners themselves and the particular experiential characteristics in the outreach site.

In contrast, the term, *identical,* refers to a narrow perception of sameness whereby the same patterns and clinical experiences are literally specified for both the on-campus and off-campus programs. Opportunity for addressing the particular learning needs of the students are restricted, for all must "march to the same drummer." It is in conceptualizing *sameness* as broader than *identical* that one can provide a dynamic, stimulating program in the outreach site that meets the needs of the learner and the community while still maintaining the integrity and quality of the program as perceived by the sponsoring agency. Essential quality controls and strategies for flexibility in meeting goals are presented in the depth discussion of the outreach program.

NEED

The recognition that need for a particular program in a designated outreach site is acknowledged, but the dimensions of that need must be considered so that the data obtained are relevant and useful in assessing the readiness of the region for such a program. The concept of need has a qualitative as well as a quantitative connotation; both must be accounted for in the decision to move the program into an off-campus location.

Acceptance by Community

Acceptance by the community and its professionals is essential for a facilitative relationship which leads to a successful experience in offering a program. The threat of an "outsider institution" coming into the area and disrupting its values and usual processes is a reality which must be acknowledged. This is particularly true if a sponsoring institution in a large metropolitan area seeks to offer a program in an out-state rural area. Invitation to the region by local representatives of the profession is a positive device, whether initiated by the residents themselves or following the sponsoring institution's notification of availability if residents are interested. The imposition of a program in a region without invitation by residents provokes many difficulties leading to lack of cooperation, support, and trust.

For each site in which the College of Nursing offered a Master of Science in Nursing degree, a request had been received for the program by the nurses in the community. In each site, nurses had completed their own assessment of the number of master's prepared nurses, the available pool of bachelor prepared nurses, and the number of nurses interested in entering such a program. The initiative shown by the regional nurses prompted consideration of their request by the college through follow-up meetings in the area and the search for funds. Obviously not all requests from various regions could be granted; they received consideration, but the final decision recognized other variables such as evidence of a mass population, geographical distribution in the state so as to equalize accessibility, community support, and access to the region by various modes of transportation. The latter is an important consideration in a state like Michigan where winter weather and distances may limit automobile travel.

Another key factor in community acceptance is the presence of significant professionals who provide leadership in mobilizing the professionals and in gaining access to the resources of the community. These individuals are most valuable in guiding the assessment and development processes so that activities are in accord with community value systems and thus are acceptable and perceived as contributing to the community welfare.

Employment Patterns

The assessment of present patterns of employment of professionals in the region provides clues as to the direction such a program should follow. Assessment considers not only the ongoing patterns, but projected patterns as health care needs change. Evidence of positions compatible with those for which the program will provide preparation and which are currently filled with less prepared individuals suggests the appropriateness of offering the program. Representatives of the sponsoring agency may also see future demands for specifically prepared professionals which are not yet evident to those in the community.

The existence of a program for preparing individuals at an advanced level may enable local agencies to upgrade the quality of preparation required for positions. In one site where the College of Nursing brought a program, the administrator of the local educational institution announced that since the faculty would now have access to a graduate program, the requirement of a master's degree in nursing would be in place at the termination of the outreach program. Because of the geographical isolation of that region, it was not realistic previously to make this requirement.

The examination of employment patterns should note those fields or positions for which employment of the graduates would be least likely to occur. In one setting, there were few public health nursing agencies with options for employment. The home care agencies wanted to employ clinical specialist practitioners. Therefore, the College of Nursing did not offer a graduate program in community health nursing, but instead emphasized clinical nursing specialties. The expense in bringing a program to an outreach region which prepares individuals for positions least available presently or projected for the future is not justified and would result in frustration for the graduates who often have limited mobility options to seek employment elsewhere.

Health Demographics

A community health profile provides data as to the clinical emphasis of programs which are designed to meet the needs of the practicing health professionals. Most health service agencies in a region are excellent resources for morbidity and mortality data. A community with a high incidence of chronic illness, infant mortality, or trauma suggests the type of clinical expertise required of the health care providers. The significant age group(s) of residents provide data for anticipating the types of health concerns and problems which one might encounter in the area.

In addition to information on illness incidence, data regarding health care delivery resources are essential in determining patterns of health care, groups responsible for the administration and delivery of services, and the resources available for clinical experiences of the professionals in the program. Some communities may have small community hospitals as the primary health service while others may be a tertiary care center for surrounding communities. Care may be provided primarily through fee for service, it may be provided through specialized groups such as health maintenance organizations (HMO) or a combination of payment systems may be in operation. The mode by which the health care needs for a community are met and the locus of decision making relative to processes and procedures used are important information in determining the need for a particular program in an area and the potential for its success.

A review of the need for a program also must consider the socioeconomic factors that characterize a community. Major sources of employment are significant for identifying the lifestyles, economic status, values, and potential health-related problems and behavior patterns. Some communities may be predominately rural, others may be semirural with one or two major employers, while others may be the major city in the region with diversity in age groups, ethnic representation, employment, and education. Knowledge about a community, its values, people, health and educational resources, and the way people work and live within some concept of health is important in determining the need for programs or parts of programs.

AVAILABILITY OF STUDENTS

In decisions relative to extending a degree program to an outreach site, the availability of candidates is a critical concern. Unfortunately, in some instances, it is the only data source used to justify a need. The number of students that are required to make a program economically feasible is a determination made by the sponsoring agency. Costs of an outreach program are considerably more than for an on-campus program, and these extra costs must be accounted for in determining minimal and maximal size of the student group that can be accommodated. Cost issues are developed in depth later in this presentation.

A general information meeting about a pending program in a community usually draws a large attendance. The size can be misleading, however, for approximately 50 percent of those individuals present will follow through with the admission process. A large number of initially interested persons is essential in order to obtain a reasonable number of students for the program. Although many attendees are sincerely interested, there also will be some who are present out of curiosity or to "hear what is said." Some individuals are not ready for the self-discipline which the program requires, especially in regard to a graduate program, nor are they prepared for the commitment necessary and the demands the program makes on their time. Some applicants have prerequisites to meet before entering the program—a perceived hurdle which some are willing to overcome while others do not have the will to persevere.

Academic Requisites

The matter of academic credentials for entering a program, particularly a graduate program, is of concern in considering the availability of students for a particular outreach program. One goal for entering out-state regions with a health professional program is to assist residents to meet requisite competencies for their area of practice when local access or individual mobility limitations are significant deterrent factors. These same factors have also effected the undergraduate preparation experienced by some applicants and thus they may not meet the academic entry requirements for graduate study.

Quality control entails admission requirements for off-campus students which are the same as for on-campus students. If a mechanism exists on campus for assisting students to meet deficits and validate their knowledge base for entering graduate study, the same mechanism can be used in the outreach site. Should such a mechanism not exist and no other accommodations are made, then the availability of a potential student body may be too limited in spite of other aspects of the projected need for such a program.

Graduate programs in nursing require for entry a bachelor's degree with a major in nursing from a National League for Nursing accredited school or college of nursing. Some schools have a system which enables those applicants not meeting the academic prerequisite to validate their nursing knowledge. The system may entail end-of-course examinations with credits allocated accordingly, course equivalency, or the use of standardized tests on the same principle as the College Level Entrance Program (CLEP) examinations in general education. The latter may be used to account for knowledge of specific undergraduate nursing courses or they may be used as a basis for determining the applicant's knowledge as it pertains to graduate study.

The sponsoring institution of a graduate nursing program needs to address the issue of prerequisites before entering regions where no accredited baccalaureate nursing program exists. Often the individuals in the region who have the appropriate academic preparation are those who moved to the area after completing the degree requirements. Many nurses in these areas completed baccalaureate degrees after graduating from a technical nursing program in whatever disciplines local institutions offered that seemed somehow related to nursing. It is not uncommon to see nurses in leadership positions in the community whose baccalaureate degree is in an area outside the field of nursing. Lacking access to an approved program or lack of mobility to go elsewhere, they were sufficiently motivated to address their perceived educational deficit through whatever means were possible.

A sensitive political issue presents itself in these circumstances. Highly respected nurse leaders in the community who lack essential academic requirements for entry into a graduate nursing program coming into the area may well have some staff members who are immediately eligible for this advanced study and preparation in their field. If a program denies access to the first group without providing realistic options for addressing deficits, yet accepts the second group, what implications does the action have on acceptance of the program in the community and the support needed to maintain it? A further question to be raised relates to the original intent of the outreach program to prepare local professionals so that they are qualified to meet the demands of their field. Does the program have anything to offer those nurses already in leadership positions who are not appropriately prepared?

The College of Nursing did have a mechanism on campus for managing the prerequisite issue which was available for use in the outreach site for those who wished to avail themselves of the options. An individual evaluation of each record in light of the college criteria identified deficits in both nursing and general education. A standardized testing program based on a baccalaureate level of nursing knowledge and decision-making skills provided data as to the applicant's readiness to pursue graduate study in nursing. General education deficits were met in local institutions of higher learning. Table 3 lists by geographic location the level of academic preparation of graduate respondent and current students.

Table 3
Baccalaureate Preparation of 154 Graduate
Respondents and 68 Current Students

Program	Acc. Bac.		Non-Acc. Bac.		Non-Nurs. Bac.		Total
	No.	%	No.	%	No.	%	
Upper Peninsula	19	70	5	19	3	11	27
Western Michigan	32	63	2	4	17	33	51
HSA VI	29	66	6	14	9	20	44
HSA VII	21	66	6	19	5	15	32
HSA III (students)	52	77	1	1	15	22	68
Total	153	69	20	9	49	22	222

The entry baccalaureate preparation of the 154 graduate respondents was: accredited baccalaureate in nursing program 66 percent (101), nonaccredited baccalaureate program in nursing 12 percent (19), and non-nursing baccalaureate program 2.2 percent (32). About two-thirds of the graduates of the outreach program met the major entry criterion: accredited baccalaureate preparation in nursing. In the present group of students, the percentage is much higher, 77 percent. Changes resulting in the increased availability of accredited baccalaureate programs in nursing within the state of Michigan are altering the profile of applicants seeking admission to graduate programs both on and off campus. Although the issue of inappropriate academic credentials for entering graduate programs is decreasing in significance, a group of older applicants who need special consideration will remain. It is essential that faculty deliberations and decisions relative to an acceptable approach to academic credentials occur prior to determining the available pool of students for an off-campus site.

Work Patterns and Family Demands

Many individuals who seek entry into the outreach program must maintain full employment, continue with designated family and community roles, and still assume the student role. The profile of graduates and students in the College of Nursing outreach programs reflect these characteristics of adults already much involved in careers and other responsibilities.

Employment at Time of Entry into the Program

At the time of entry into the graduate nursing program, 95 percent (144) of the graduate respondents and 96 percent (65) of the present students were employed. The analysis of the positions these individuals held yields support for the previous statement that many potential students already hold positions for which they are unprepared. Table 4 illustrates positions of graduate respondents and current students at their time of entry into the program.

Four of these positions, faculty, administrator (including supervisor), in-service educator and clinical specialist, are considered appropriate for individuals with a minimum of a master's degree. Among the graduate respondents, 73 percent (111) were employed in these positions at the time they entered the program. Note that the largest percentage (43) were faculty in schools of nursing. There were 25 individuals (17 percent) who were employed as staff nurses, the generally accepted area of practice for a nurse with a baccalaureate degree preparation.

Although the current group of students has a larger percentage (31) of nurses who were employed as staff nurses at the time of entry to the program, there is still a large percentage (62) who are in leadership positions.

A further analysis of these data examined entry employment of two groups of students, those who met the requisite academic preparation criterion and those who did not (see Table 5). The data support the previously made statement that many individuals who do not meet this criterion are already employed in leadership positions.

Leadership positions requiring a minimum of master's preparation in nursing were held at the time of entry into the program by 86 percent (44) of those whose baccalaureate was not from an accredited program while 73 percent (67) of those meeting the criterion were in these positions. The latter group had more employed in staff nurse positions, 20 percent (20) than did the former group, 10 percent (5).

The profile of students who enter a graduate professional program would probably not differ significantly from what the College of Nursing found as it entered areas where access to accredited baccalaureate programs in nursing is limited for residents. The question of how to meet the community need for qualified persons in leadership positions must take into account these individuals who do not have the requisite preparation for entry into an advanced program. It can generally be acknowledged that

Table 4
Positions of Graduate Respondents and Current Students at Time of Entry into Program

Positions Held	Graduates		Students	
	No.	%	No.	%
Faculty	66	43	17	25
Administrator	19	13	8	12
Staff nurse	25	17	21	31
In-service educator	15	10	5	7
Clinical specialist	6	4	2	3
Supervisor	5	3	10	15
Unemployed	8	5	2	3
Other	8	5	3	4
Total	152	100	68	100

Table 5
Baccalaureate Criterion for Graduate Respondents in
Leadership Position at Time of Entry into Program

Position	Baccalaureate Criterion Met		Baccalaureate Criterion Not Met	
	No.	%	No.	%
Faculty	39	39	27	52
Administrator	14	14	10	20
In-service educator	10	10	5	10
Clinical specialist	4	4	2	4
Total	101	73	44	86

these nurses will remain in these positions whether or not they are accepted into the program.

The College of Nursing through its own mechanism was able to provide options for those who did not meet the major academic criterion and admitted them to the program. These nurses were then brought into the mainstream of nursing education and were prepared to continue in their leadership positions with the needed advanced preparation.

The issue of working student population influences the decision as to whether a full-time or part-time program will be needed. Definitions of a full-time or part-time student are in accord with the specific policies of the sponsoring agency. A significant consideration in planning is the number of credits that a student, particularly one who is employed, can expect to enroll for in a given term, particularly if the term includes laboratory or clinical practice courses.

Although at some periods in the program students may take a leave of absence or decrease work time, this option seems less available. Recession in Michigan occurred after the initiation of the outreach master's program. Many of the students needed to work full-time being the sole breadwinner in the family. Current students are encountering another barrier for the use of options to provide for more time for the program due to social pressures to decrease health care costs. The tightening of the labor market in nursing has meant that if nurses take an educational leave or a decrease in working time, they are vulnerable to loss of their employment. A further factor is the general policy whereby educational financial assistance as a fringe benefit is allotted only to full-time employees. The high cost of education, including books, tuition, and travel, is often beyond the resources of many family budgets. Limited availability of scholarship money means that most students need to have access to the educational cost reimbursement provided by their employer.

The demands of work expectations are not the only pressure experienced by the outreach students. In the College of Nursing outreach graduate program, most of the outreach students are women, which added the demands entailed in the roles of mother and wife. Table 6 illustrates the marital status of graduate respondents and current students at entry into the program.

The present student group has a larger percent of single students, 29 percent (20) than one finds among the graduates when they entered the program, 7 percent (10). It is difficult to explain this difference, for data on age differences do not show any significance. It may be a funtion of the present trend among career women to delay marriage.

Children were reported by 118 graduates, 77 percent. The range in number was from 1 to 7 with an age range from 1 to 30.

These data would be representative of what one might expect from any student population comprising a large number of women. Although similar findings would be found relative to a male population, the demands of male roles in current society are less threatening to their ability to enter and persevere in an outreach program.

Age Distribution

Another piece of data relative to availability of students is the anticipated age of applicants. The positions they hold in employment and the community and the family responsibilities they have assumed suggest an older, more mature population than one might expect in an on-campus program. This older age may be a function of the residents' lack of access to a degree program and thus the need to defer further education. Data from the graduate outreach programs reflect this phenomenon (see Table 7).

The mean age of the graduates at the time of their entry into the program was 35.43 years. The return of the older student to academic studies is a current phenomenon. However, in nursing there is a trend whereby individuals enroll in a master's program shortly after completing their baccalaureate preparation. This means that a younger group of nurses is entering graduate study, a trend that is becoming increasingly evident as the goal of a doctorate in nursing becomes more realistic for nurses. The ages represented in this population are less typical of the current practice on the main campus. It probably reflects the lack of access and opportunity for advanced study experienced by individuals far removed from the main campus.

Other Factors

Before concluding discussion of the qualitative dimensions of student availability, two other variables must be identified. Both affect the student potential by their dependence on the type of class schedule pattern to be used. One factor relates to the cultural and religious mores in the community. In one area where the College of Nursing program was located, several potential applicants were Seventh Day Adventists who could not attend class on the weekend pattern consisting of Friday nights and Saturdays. That pattern had been developed to accommodate the larger number of students who resided outside the immediate outreach site who could not have participated if the

Table 6
Marital Status of Graduate Respondents and
Current Students at Entry into Program

Marital Status	Graduates		Students	
	No.	%	No.	%
Single	10	7	20	29
Married	128	83	44	65
Widowed	1	1	—	—
Divorced	14	9	4	6
Separated	1	1	—	—
Total	154	100	68	100

program followed the usual weekly academic calendar. The second factor addresses the recognition that availability of students for a program includes a large geographical area from which students travel into the site for the program. In one program, a graduate of the College of Nursing outreach program reported that she had traveled 16,280 miles for her master's degree.

The data relative to the outreach program of the college are typical to what one might find if a program is brought into a location where no other such program existed. Availability of potential students in determining the need for a particular off-campus program refers to much more than the number of students who express interest. The notion of availability has a qualitative dimension; that is, *who* is the potential student; for decisions as to whether or not an institution of higher learning can respond to a need is influenced by how the decision-making bodies respond to issues of prerequisites, a student body with work and family demands, an older age group of students who may not have participated in a formal educational experience for some time, and a student group that resides at a considerable distance from the main center of activities in the outreach area. Fit between student characteristics and the way the program is delivered is essential. A traditional orientation and commitment will be less likely to yield a successful program directed toward meeting the needs of a maximum number of health care professionals.

Table 7
Age Distribution of Graduate Respondents and Current
Students at Entry into Program

Age Range	Graduates		Students	
	No.	%	No.	%
20–29	35	24	18	26
30–39	69	46	30	44
40–49	41	28	18	26
50–59	4	2	2	4

COMMITMENT

The demonstrated need for an outreach program and the availability of students challenge an institution of higher learning to respond, often with enthusiasm. However, the meaning and implications of such a response relative to the nature of the commitment entailed must be examined before action is initiated. Commitment entails acceptance of the endeavor by the sponsoring institution, the school and college where the program is housed, and the faculty as a whole that is responsible for the program. Commitment is also moral and pragmatic. Potential students must be assured that if they enter the program, they will indeed be able to complete degree requirements in a quality program which offers access to and availability of all resources necessary for the program.

Moral Commitment

An institution of higher learning brings an outreach program to an off-campus site with reasonable assurance that it will remain in the area for a sufficient time to enable students to earn the designated degree. This commitment requires planning that encompasses the total program, not that which addresses start-up activities with a "wait-and-see" attitude that requires the students to come to campus to complete the degree if the program does not work. The latter solution is generally not a solution for many students whose reason for enrolling in the outreach program was because of lack of flexibility for attending a main campus program. However, provision for contingency plans is necessary to meet situations which may require program termination while some students are still enrolled.

The commitment is two-fold: it requires that the community supply sufficient students to make the outreach program educationally and economically feasible and that the sponsoring agency fulfill its responsibility to commit resources that will reasonably assure continuance of the program through the designated period of time. The commitment must be stated clearly so that both the community and the sponsoring agency acknowledge their responsibilities for maintaining the program except for unforeseen circumstances which might arise. Such a statement needs to protect the students in the program at the time from such untoward events as change in administration in the sponsoring agency, change in faculty, or lack of readiness to continue supplying needed resources.

The stated commitment pertains to the possibility of completing a program. Should some students choose to move more slowly through the program at a decreased pace than projected, the obligation of the institution to remain in the area is not relevant, for these students need to make their own arrangements to fulfill requirements. The sponsoring institution would be expected to assist these students to earn their degrees; it is the students who must make the necessary arrangements when the program leaves the area.

The core element in commitment is trust. Potential students considering entering an outreach program raise the critical questions: If I start, will I be able to finish? Will the program stay here long enough for me to finish my degree requirements? During the first two outreach programs that the College of Nursing offered, this element of trust was a factor. Students reported experiences with previous commitments by agencies that were unfulfilled; the start of courses toward a degree, but the rest of the courses never arrived; the perceived promise to bring a program to the region, again none arrived. Early in the program, anxiety which is associated with questioning trust was noted in several ways. For example, when students encountered a faculty member who was not perceived to be "thrilled" to be teaching in the outreach program, they became concerned that other faculty would not want to come and teach them. After the college completed two programs in the state and demonstrated its resolve to meet commitments, the element of trust became less a matter to be reckoned with in the other programs.

Commitment of Resources

Resources, which will be discussed more in depth in a later section, encompass financial, personnel, educational, and supportive services. Each of these resources is examined within the context of the notion of quality programming to determine the specific demands for outreach programs.

Financial resources, which account for the extraordinary costs in exporting and conducting programs in outreach locations, must be planned relative to the total time period projected for the program, not just for the start-up in the first year. Likewise, when outside grant funds are sought, the grant needs to consider, at a minimum, the costs entailed for the time necessary for one cohort of students to complete degree requirements, generally two to three years, so that financial security can be reasonably assured. Of course, unanticipated economic events may threaten the financial stability and thus the relationship between the availability of funds and the continuance of the program needs to be clearly stated to all parties concerned.

Shortly after the College of Nursing began its outreach programs, economic recession struck Michigan with force. Funding for an advanced training grant from the Division of Nursing, Department of Health and Human Resources was obtained. Since recession was a national phenomenon, federal funds for nursing were also threatened and the need arose on several occasions to develop a worse case budget and proposals for less costly programming by which the university could assist students already in the program if the outside funding was discontinued. Realistic budgeting for outreach programs with consideration of the range for minimal and maximal allocation of funds is a critical factor in making the commitment to bring a degree program into an outreach site.

Personnel commitment represents considerable financial commitment as it entails salary, travel, and other instructional costs for faculty and other support personnel such as a coordinator, secretaries, or computer operators. Commitment also addresses quality, especially in the selection of teaching personnel in accord with standards demanded by the sponsoring agency. Quality, especially in master's programs, means high cost faculty. It is in this commitment that the institution declares its obligation to offer a first class program. It is the fear of many students, and this fear has been supported by some ill-planned off-campus programs, that the faculty selected to teach will result in a diluted second class program.

Instructional resources including the environment and books, teaching materials, library, computer access, and so on, as well as the support services needed by any educational program are important factors in planning for an outreach program. As with all resources, there is both a qualitative and quantitative dimension to their allocation and the commitment the institution makes.

Although the specifics in resource allocation are not noted here, it is important that any provision for an outreach program include commitment to their allocation in accord with the requirements for a quality program.

CONCLUSION

The decision to offer an outreach program for health care providers requires analysis of five major elements: concept of quality, need for program, availability of students, availability of resources, and commitment to the program. Each of these elements is significant in assessing the appropriateness of an institution of higher learning in extending its programs to an outreach site. Each element has a qualitative and quantitative dimension.

Quality of the program assures the maintenance of the standards in the outreach site for which the on-campus program is held. It recognizes the difference between concepts of identical and sameness in the development and implementation of its design as it plans for various routes to the attainment of the program objectives to accommodate specific needs of the learners involved.

Need for a program includes the acknowledgement of such factors as community acceptance, employment patterns in the field of study for which the program prepares, health demographics in terms of morbidity, mortality, and health care resources.

Availability of students extends beyond the mere counting of a sufficient number of individuals expressing interest to incorporating decisions about requisites for entry, work patterns, and family responsibilities which place great demands on the individuals involved, age of potential students which may mean some older students who may not have participated in formal study for some time, and the inclusion of students from an extended geographical area. A sufficient number of interested individuals may be available in the community, but will the program enable them to participate?

Commitment is both moral, the reasonable assurance that students who enter the program will be able to complete degree requirements, and pragmatic in terms of allocation of financial, personnel, educative, and support resources. The decision to offer the professional program in an outreach site is not based on the notion of a "quick fix" to address enrollment or other such matters. It is a serious deliberative process with many ramifications for the sponsoring institution during and long after the program ceases.

3

Design of a Quality Outreach Program:
The Community-Based Model

A model of an educational program is a structural design which depicts inter-relationships among various component parts. Specifically, a model of an outreach program is a visual representation of the organizational structure which serves as a framework for operational decisions throughout the existence of the program.

There are multiple models for outreach programs, each one based on certain philosophical notions and assumptions about educational programs as well as the organizational and institutional policies and patterns particular to the sponsoring institution. Some models may be replicated in various institutions; some may require modifications to accommodate specific policies of an institution, whereas some may be unique to a particular institution's pattern of delivery of educational programs or the uniqueness of the outreach location.

Model development is guided by principles which assure quality controls in all program aspects so that the integrity of the on-campus program is maintained in the outreach site. It provides for adherence to policies and standards by which decision-making processes are guided. It designates the locus of accountability for the selection and allocation of resources in accord with program needs and the guidelines specified in the institution's policies and procedures.

MODELS BASED ON BELIEFS REGARDING SOCIALIZATION

How much of the program for preparing health care providers should be offered off campus? Is there something special about educational experiences on campus that requires all students to participate to some degree in these experiences? In the health care provider fields, much concern is expressed about the need to socialize students into designated professional roles and modes of behavior. Can this socialization occur in a total outreach program or must students spend time in the campus environment to achieve this end?

Responses to the above questions reflect faculty philosophical beliefs about the educational process which in turn influence the model of the outreach program. Some models of outreach programs provide for total experience to be conducted in the outreach site with the belief that there are other mechanisms for promoting socialization. This model accepts the basic reason for the outreach program, the limited mobility option for the students, thus necessitating that the entire program be available in the designated area. The community resources are maximized to provide the clinical practice necessary for meeting the stated competency level objectives. Library and other resources are supplemented as needed to enable students to have access to the essential literature in their fields.

Some models provide for parts of the program to be offered in the outreach site while others carry the requisite that the students attend classes on campus. The selection of the curriculum component(s) for which students must come to campus is a decision of the faculty based on its beliefs about requirements for achieving specific objectives. One graduate program in nursing proposed conducting all nonclinical nursing courses in the outreach site and required all students to attend clinical courses on campus and gain practice experience in the health care facilities used by on-campus students. The egocentrism reflected by this decision raises questions about the faculty's commitment to the health care of the community where they are offering their program. In other models students go to the main campus for one or two courses so as to share learning experiences with on-campus students and access the resources of the college/university.

Another type of on-campus experience incorporated in some models is not directly related to the course structure in the program. It involves a brief experience, a weekend or perhaps a week, which is directed more toward socialization. The planned program generally entails seminars with on-campus students and faculty, tour of the campus facilities, and a social event for sharing ideas in an informal setting.

Except for the first model, there is a basic belief of the faculty that students need some type of contact with students, faculty, and resources of the institution from which they will receive their degree. The intensity and nature of the contact reflects beliefs about the significance of on-campus experience to the learning process and the means by which professional socialization develops. In the first model where all learning experiences are conducted in the outreach site, decisions of faculty reflect a different notion about the learning process and the attainment of professionalization. This model requires a creative approach to program development so as to draw on the resources of the community and the school sponsoring the offering.

MODELS BASED ON OPERATIONAL STRUCTURE

Models reflect not only faculty's beliefs about where learning and socialization occur, but also the structural relationship of the outreach program and the sponsoring institution.

Satellite Centers

Satellite centers have been established by some institutions of higher learning in communities removed from the main campus. These centers are integrated organizationally in the institution's framework with a staff identified as employees of that institution. These centers are financially supported by the parent institution and provide support services for the schools/colleges who use them for off-campus programs. The institutional units who use the centers are often responsible for meeting the costs of their particular staff and may be expected to meet the costs for office facilities. Classrooms and instructional resources in the center are shared by all programs since the costs are included in the center's budget. Faculty who conduct outreach programs for health care providers access the resources of the center and have the advantage of entering a community which already accepts programs from the sponsoring institution. The major responsibilities of these colleges/universities is the selection of a director of the program for coordination purposes, providing for faculty, and arranging for use of the community resources as needed for the program. Teaching staff may represent on-campus faculty coming to the center, appointment of qualified individuals in the area as faculty, or a combination of both.

Partnership

In this model, the operation of the outreach program is a shared enterprise with the sponsoring institution of higher learning and another institution in the community. This arrangement usually involves sharing resources, including costs of the program. The responsibility for program quality and decisions affecting the conduct of the educational program reside within the educational institution offering the degree. Several examples of this model exist. In some regions, Area Health Education Centers (AHEC) share in the operation of degree programs in outreach sites. A partnership exists between the University of North Carolina at Greensboro School of Nursing and the Northwest Area Health Education Center of Winston-Salem, North Carolina, in offering a Bachelor of Science in Nursing degree program in that region. The university is fully responsible for the quality of the program and the appointment of the teaching staff. Northwest AHEC provides office space and support services to the director and assists in meeting the extraordinary costs entailed in the outreach program.

A different organizational relationship exists between the University of California at San Francisco and Stanford University Hospital in offering a Master of Science in Nursing degree. Stanford University Hospital assumes a significant portion of the financial costs, including the director of the program and her office and staff, instructional facilities, and support services and faculty. Prepared nurses in the hospital receive adjunct appointments from the university for their teaching responsibilities in the program. The program itself is the same one offered on campus by the School of Nursing in the university. These are only two examples of the partnership model. Other modifications exist. The significant factor in this model is the existence of an agency in the outreach site with the resources to assist the educational institution to meet the extraordinary costs of outreach programs through both financial and in-kind contributions.

Interinstitutional Model

In this model, two educational institutions offering a degree program for the preparation of the same type of health care professional form a cooperative arrangement for bringing an outreach program to an off-campus site. This model was developed by the Medical College of Virginia and the University of Virginia in providing for a master's degree in nursing in two outreach locations in Virginia. The goal of the project was to strengthen and expand graduate education in nursing in the state through interuniversity cooperation and collaboration. This model provides an opportunity for sharing limited resources, especially in relation to prepared faculty, and for distributing costs. It is a less frequently used model than other types, for the commitment to cooperation often involves matters such as institutional identity, discrepancies in program and degree requirements, the decision as to which institution awards the degree, and vested interests.

Other Models

Numerous other models for outreach programming exist. The University of Alabama, Birmingham, developed a model for bringing a Master of Science in Nursing degree to four sites in the state where such an opportunity was lacking. This model entailed cooperation with institutions of higher learning and health care facilities in the regions as resources for the program. Unlike the partnership model, monies from several budgets toward the cost of the program were not allocated; the contributions were primarily in-kind. As described by Kelley and Flowers (1985), faculty costs were by the university which sent on-campus faculty into the region for major teaching responsibilities.

Another model, used by the University of Michigan for its outreach baccalaureate program, has the university assuming the major cost for the program. An on-site office is located in the region, usually rented in one of the educational institutions.

COMMUNITY-BASED MODEL

The College of Nursing, Wayne State University, developed a community-based model which it used in all its outreach programs leading to a Master of Science in Nursing degree. When the College of Nursing received a request from nurses in the outreach site to bring the graduate program to their areas, it considered the impact such an endeavor could have on the community's ability to deliver health care services to its constituents. The decision to provide an outreach program must involve the recognition that its effect can extend beyond that which involves the individuals in the program or the profession. Initially, to the first request, the college decided to offer a one time program, staying in the region until one cohort of students had the opportunity to complete degree requirements.

Model for Total Degree Program

The model most appropriate for the College of Nursing to make the greatest impact on nursing and health care in the outreach community provided for the total program to be brought to the area. The decision not to provide a program requiring both on-campus and off-campus experiences recognized that the primary student population would consist of employed married women with children whose mobility was somewhat restricted. A further deterrent to this option was the inability of the health care agencies in the community to relinquish their limited nursing resources for any extended period of time.

The full program model makes it possible for a large number of nurses to be prepared at one time without too much disruption of service to the local community. This approach, a one time full program offering, provides for a "mass inoculation" of a community which facilitates its ability to make changes in health care practices through several mechanisms. When a large number of individuals are in the same program, they share experiences in exploring together various theories, intervening variables, and proposals for resolution of problems. This interaction promotes a collegial support group system for instituting and addressing change issues. A network is established providing for a valuable resource to the individuals as they continue their own professional growth. The continuing significance of this network has been cited by some graduates in their questionnaire returns. For example:

> I also am grateful to have found my community colleagues and the support that that brings.

I feel more enjoyment in the profession of nursing after having completed the MSN program. I suppose a lot of this is because of the many new relationships with nursing colleagues and with other health care providers.

Self-image was good, but is enhanced related to extensive educational program, professional linkage with peers in the program.

The use of health care facilities in the community for clinical practice experience in the program becomes a significant means of initiating change as new ideas are introduced by the learners in the setting. Some students in the program were asked by the director of nursing in some agencies to present a conference to their staffs about a new concept they were learning and possibly having an experience within the practice setting. Some students had clinical experience in the agencies where they were employed and thus were acceptable to the staff when introducing new ideas. Agencies involved in the learning process are more likely to support change than when a graduate from outside the region tries to introduce a new idea or practice which is generally unknown in the local community. In this type of model, it is the faculty who are outsiders, and they must assume responsibility to function within the cultural and social mores of the community. Concepts, ideas, and problem solutions are examined within the context of the community mores and those of the institutions involved. The resident students provide the framework for discussion and interpretation and then serve as change agents. Maintaining practice experience in the outreach site is an enriching experience for the community and for the faculty. The faculty has the opportunity to examine ideas in a setting different from those associated with the on-campus program and thus continue their own professional growth.

The decision to offer the full nursing program in the outreach site required that the college develop a model to address the question: How can it provide for this influx of change in a community far removed from campus with a minimum cost to the university, faculty, and students in terms of money and energy output while maintaining the same quality program that was being offered on campus. The design of the model was influenced by the intent of the college to offer a one time Master of Science in Nursing program, thus no capital investment was indicated. There would be no "turf" declaration, no issue of territory, no real threat to the community of continued presence in the area suggesting take over by the out-state educational institution. It was also recognized that the college might offer such a program in other regions, so that the model developed needed to be transferable.

Assumptions Relative to the Outreach Program

Certain assumptions about the outreach program were stated as a basis for preparing the model:

The degree program must be requested by the community itself.

The program will be offered only if there is no other institution in the area providing a similar program.

Because the program is on an outreach basis, it must be maintained on its own budget.

Attempts would be made to keep student tuition at the same amount as that stated for on-campus students. Funding for the extraordinary costs of faculty travel and administrative expenses entailed with maintaining a program so far off campus would be sought.

The program must be self-supporting financially.

The commitment of the College of Nursing would be maintained as long as the costs were being met and there were sufficient quantities of students. The college would guarantee students in the program the opportunity to complete degree requirements.

The total program is under the control of Wayne State University and must meet the same standards and requirements of the graduate programs in the College of Nursing.

Appointment of faculty other than those from the College of Nursing would be in accord with policies and procedures of the university and the particular college.

The program must provide for use of resources (facilities and people) already in the designated area, so that the university provides only those services that are not available in the region.

The relationship between the university and the community is a reciprocal, supportive one.

Criteria of the Model

The community-based model for the Master of Science in Nursing Outreach Program is required to meet the following criteria:

It must be consistent with the goals and values of the community.

It must maintain the educational integrity of the courses and the total program offered on campus.

It must show cost effectiveness.

It must be flexible to provide for innovation in design and implementation of courses and the total program.

It must be designed to be feasible and convenient for participants and faculty.

It must provide for the reciprocal relationship between the university and the community.

It must lend itself to evaluation.

Description of the Model

The community-based model is represented by four interlocking cir-cles with communication avenues among the four. Each circle represents one of the contributing components to the program. Figure 2 illustrates the community-based model.

Community.

It provides a location to serve as a base of operations for schedul-ing all activities of the program. (This is an in-kind contribution.)

It provides access to media (newspapers, TV stations) for sharing information with the community, potential students, and students.

It provides for a vital link between community residents and groups, the students, the College of Nursing, and Wayne State University.

It provides an advisory group of nursing leaders and students for direction and feedback to the college, thus permitting responsive-ness to shared concerns.

Figure 2
Community-Based Model

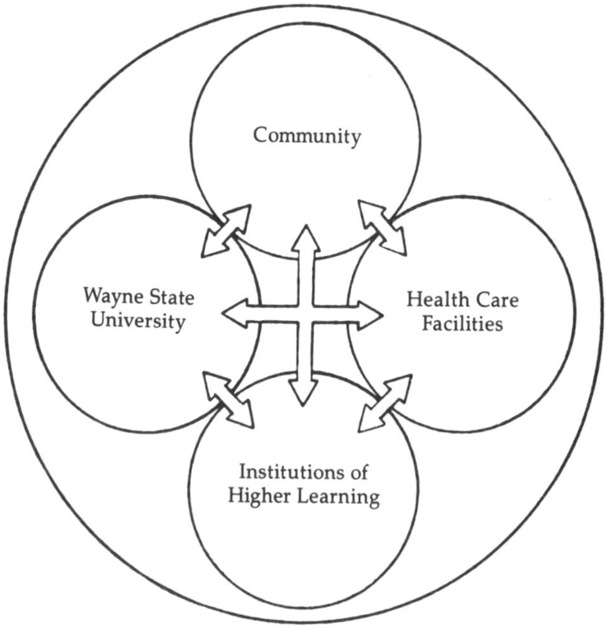

It provides library resources, book stores, instructional and meeting facilities, as well as any other support services needed.

Wayne State University College of Nursing.

It maintains responsibility for decision making in regard to all components of the program.

It receives all student applications, assesses records, accepts applicants to the program, and awards degrees.

It has absolute control over all faculty teaching. The College of Nursing provides faculty for all nursing courses either from its own group or through contracts with qualified persons in the community.

It approves all non-nursing courses offered by community universities in consultation with appropriate Wayne State University departments. The appropriate department in Wayne State University approves an individual within the community to teach one of Wayne's non-nursing courses when the course is not available in the community.

It plans programs and schedules courses and classes to keep student and faculty travel within reasonable limits. A pattern of clinical courses on one weekend and functional or research courses on the alternate weekend has proven most effective.

It provides coordinators for each clinical nursing department to give academic counseling.

It monitors the quality of program throughout the year through department meetings and periodic outreach advisory committee meetings.

It provides for consultation between faculty and the community, thus facilitating infusion of data.

It carries out a systematic evaluation of the total program.

Health Care Facilities in the Community.

They provide opportunities for practice components of the program and available space for individual and group conferences.

They recommend to the College of Nursing that clinical nursing practitioners assist in teaching.

They provide in-kind contributions, such as libraries, the instructional materials necessary for teaching, classrooms, and meeting space.

Institutions of Higher Learning in the Community.

They provide in-kind contributions, such as classroom space, use of library and learning resources, facilitation of book purchasing mechanisms, and use of hardware for multimedia presentations.

They provide cognate courses required in the program; thus, this program generates student credit hours for the local institutions.

They often provide low-cost housing for students who come into the region for weekend classes.

They assist in the identification of potential faculty to teach a Wayne State University cognate course when such a course is not available in the area.

APPLICATION OF THE COMMUNITY-BASED MODEL

The community-based model, developed during the first outreach program and used in all subsequent programs, has served most effectively as a framework for decision making and allocation of responsibility and accountability.

In all settings, the community-based model was most effective in meeting the objective to offer a total Master of Science in Nursing Outreach Program in underserved areas of the state. The model prevented duplication of efforts and resources, contributed to the educational institutions in the region, and mobilized the resources available from the community. As a result, the College of Nursing was able to concentrate much of its teaching efforts on the nursing component of the program. At the conclusion of the program, the College of Nursing was able to withdraw from the community, leaving behind a group of well-prepared nurses, but no buildings or other capital investments.

In each site, there was a group of key nurse leaders who facilitated the college's entry into the community, often by introducing the director of the outreach program to significant individuals in the community who could assist in mobilizing the needed resources. Some of these leaders became core persons in the formulation of the community advisory committee which provided assistance and support throughout the time the program was in the area.

On-Site Office

The distance to the outreach site from the main campus necessitated a locus of operations in the area which would be the main center serving the needs of the program, faculty, and students. Such a facility with all the essential support services is readily available to programs whose sponsoring institution has satellite centers in the region. When a program is new to an area and the only one from that particular institution of higher learning, an on-site office must be procured.

Several considerations were entailed in determining the selection of an office for the nursing program.

Space needs required two offices to accommodate the coordinator and the secretary with provision for a conference area to be used by faculty and students. Additional space was required when a computer and word processor were purchased for use by the staff and students.

The office needed to be located in a neutral site so that the program would maintain its identity as a Wayne State University offering. Direct association with an institution where a nursing program already exists or with a hospital runs the risk of the program being perceived as belonging to that agency or serving the particular needs of that agency. A suggestion of such a possibility was made when one institution of higher learning offered office facilities on its campus with the reminder that the real purpose of the College of Nursing outreach program was to help the institution develop its own master's program. Since the intent of the college was to serve all nurses in the region, the need for an on-site office in a neutral location was evident.

The site needed to be in close proximity to where classes were held so that it could be readily available to faculty and students when they came into the region for class.

Since the program was to be a one time event, no major financial investment in the office and its equipment could be made.

The allocation of office space and utilities as well as major furnishings would need to be in-kind contributions if the program was to be cost effective and the goal of maintaining tuition within on-campus rates was to be met. This consideration was of major significance since the programs continued through a period of severe recession in Michigan.

In all four sites, including the present site, the community provided space and essential furnishings for an on-site office. In the first site, office and staff were provided for in the Upper Peninsula Comprehensive Health Planning Office. The experiences in this office contributed to the refinement of the community-based model by providing knowledge as to the planning needed. The second site had office space in the University Consortium, a center developed by all institutions in the state who offered courses or other educational experiences in Western Michigan. Although Wayne State University was not a member of this consortium, the College of Nursing was graciously welcomed and provided with office facilities.

The third program was located in the Mid-Michigan Area Health Education Center based on the grounds of Veterans Hospital. A very different arrangement was made for the fourth site with headquarters in Traverse City. A community leader who saw the outreach program as benefiting the health care of the community donated space in an unused office he owned. Major furnishings were provided by Northwestern Michigan College and the accountant of the donor. The current program is located in a small house on the property of Borgess Medical Center in Kalamazoo.

The college purchased limited equipment for the offices such as files, typewriter, conference table, and the usual desk supplies. In each location after the first one, the college assumed cost for the several telephone lines needed for office use. When the computers were purchased, the college provided the necessary tables, storage facilities, etc. The limitations in equipment purchases greatly facilitated the closure process of the office and the opening of a new one in another site as well as keeping moving costs to a minimum.

The in-kind contribution of an office and appropriate facilities was a major one and will be discussed in a later chapter on costs. Such generosity was reflective of the recognition that this type of graduate program was new to the area and that it had much to contribute to the education of nurses and the development of health care services within the community.

Instructional Resources

Classroom. In all programs, in-kind contributions for instructional resources were most generously offered. Because the program was a one time event in each community, institutions of higher learning readily made classroom space available: Northern Michigan University and Lake Superior College in the Upper Peninsula; Nazareth College, Mercy Hospital School of Nursing, and Grand Rapids Community College in the Western Michigan program; Saginaw Valley College and Delta Community College in HSA VI; and Northwestern Community College and North Central Community College in HSA VII. In the current program, classes are held in the educational center at Bronson Hospital and at Borgess Medical Center.

All the facilities had sufficient multimedia hardware for use by faculty and students in classroom settings. In several settings, the college rented video cameras for a course that related history taking and physical examination.

Book Purchasing

Books required for courses were ordered and distributed by bookstores in the region, especially those in institutions of higher learning when possible. In one instance, a local bookstore in a community served as a resource. The order for required books was given to the responsible person in the bookstore and students purchased books on site. In one setting, personnel from the bookstore brought books to the first class of the term so that the students could purchase them at that time. Bookstore hours are of major concern when students travel into a site for early evening or weekend classes. It is essential that planning assure student access to the bookstore at the beginning of the term.

The system by which book purchasing was maintained in the on-site region has its logistic merits, but also it is a valuable strategy for maintaining good will in the community. The financial gains in book purchases are kept within the community and the students' use of the bookstore extends to purchases beyond the books. The system has been most effective for all the outreach programs, although the rapid rise of book costs in the past few years has been unsettling to students.

This cost issue was a major factor and the only real difficulty which the college encountered in implementing this system. In one course, students complained about the high price of a required text. Responding sympathetically, the instructor made the purchase of the book optional which then resulted in few purchases. The bookstore director called the program director expressing concern that a large number of a required text was still on the shelf and they were going to be returned. The cost of handling and returning the books now had to be borne by the bookstore.

Faculty on campus seldom are concerned about the number of books they order and the number purchased except when supply does not meet student demand. However, when seeking the services of an off-campus agency, it is important to be as accurate as possible in determining a book order. Professional books are generally specific to a particular population and have little sale potential to others who use the bookstore services. The cost of handling the books needs to be met by the purchase of the books.

Library

Library resources are a critical component of any higher education experience. Availability and access to the literature in the field are major concerns in providing educational experiences in outreach sites. The issue is a serious one when graduate programs are being offered in sites where graduate programs are minimal.

The community-based model provides for use of all libraries in the region; in institutions of higher learning, health care agencies, and local library systems. A major assessment of all holdings in books, periodicals, and monographs is necessary to determine resources relevant to the need of the program. In this regard, conferences with librarians responsible for each library to be used are essential so that librarians understand program needs and the program understands the extent of resources available.

Library services in all outreach programs were provided as in-kind contributions except during a period in one program. During the first year of that program, students were enrolled in a course concerned with history taking and physical assessment. The course was self-paced and required use of multiple slide-tapes which the library staff housed and distributed to the students in addition to their service regarding books, periodicals, and so on. A nominal sum of money was given to the library during the two terms that course was taught in recognition of the extra demand being placed on the library staff.

Specific libraries were designated as main sources of material. Because of the widespread geographical distribution of students for each program, it was necessary to identify from two to four libraries as major sources. The identification was based on the location of a critical mass of students. For example, in the HSA VII program, Traverse City was the locus of operations and thus Northwestern Michigan College provided library services. Because of the geographical location of students, libraries were located in three other locations: Petoskey, Big Rapids, and Sault Ste. Marie. The on-site office also became a locus of reference books purchased and mimeographed articles, especially for individual students who did not have ready access to any of the designated libraries. These individuals were able to borrow the reference material from the office and return it by mail if necessary.

The procedure for assuring availability of library resources was followed in most settings. The bibliography for each course was sent to the on-site coordinator who checked with the libraries to determine what required holdings were available. The newsletter to the students noted the location of references if they were not generally distributed.

A major concern related to those references which were not available to students in the outreach site. This matter is especially crucial in graduate education since the regions where these outreach programs were located had no graduate program in nursing. Several approaches to resolving this matter are available to program planners. Interlibrary loan systems are certainly a viable option. Temporary transfer of selected references from the main campus to the outreach site is another mechanism. The difficulty with this system is that often the same course is being offered at the same time both on campus and off campus. Libraries generally do not have sufficient copies of a reference to supply students in two sites. In the past few years, a complication has arisen with the great influx of new reference books in nursing and related fields representing new authors and new editions. While faculty chose to use these new references, many libraries had not yet incorporated them into their holdings.

Experience in outreach programs convinced planners that the most effective way to address this matter is by direct purchase of reference books to put on reserve in designated libraries. Allocation for book purchases also needs to be an item in the outreach budget. In most instances a copy of a book was purchased for each designated library and for the on-site office. However, if students registered in a particular course requiring a specific book did not reside in an area of one of the libraries, then fewer copies were purchased.

Access to professional magazines may or may not be an issue. Such an issue could arise if the magazine is from a discipline other than nursing or one generally used in graduate programs. When a magazine issue has several required articles, such as often occurs with *Advances in Nursing Science*, the students may purchase the issue or copies of the issue may be purchased for reserve in each of the appropriate libraries. The need to duplicate articles is an expectation when offering programs, especially graduate programs, in the outreach site. The plan that proved most effective for this program was for the college to duplicate articles, stamp them with the appropriate copyright message, and distribute to the designated libraries and the on-site office. In the various libraries, the students had access to copying facilities should they desire to make their own personal copies. This practice of copying occurred frequently since the students traveled considerable distances for the program and usually combined work, family responsibility, and student role. Time budgeted for reading was not always compatible with scheduled library hours. When tapes were used as resource to courses, they too were distributed to the appropriate libraries and access to a viewing machine was provided by the library staff. Within the libraries, the staff was most helpful to students doing library searches such as Medline and to obtain references not within the holdings of the library.

Continuous care and concern about the library needs of the program is an important matter throughout the entire program. One factor that caused some difficulty in using on-site libraries involved the scheduled library hours. Often the institution where the library was located used different vacation and holiday schedules than did Wayne State University. Library hours during the Christmas holiday period were often restricted or nonexistent in community colleges, unlike what occurs on a university campus. Efforts were made to notify students of the library schedule so that they could plan accordingly.

For the most part, the system for meeting the library resources worked well. In the first program, a difficulty arose when the librarian in one school chose that summer to have all the editions of *Nursing Research* bound. Although this was a fine decision for the institution, it was most disadvantageous for the program since that was the term in which the nursing research course was taught. A set of faculty copies was quickly dispersed to the library for reserve holding. The necessity of notifying the librarian in the community relative to anticipated needs was made evident.

In general, the students were satisfied with the system developed, although they sometimes evidenced a distorted perception of the easy access on-campus students have to library materials. A greater variety of the literature in the field does exist on campus, but direct access to required materials was more available to outreach students. When students needed a resource not readily available off campus, the on-campus staff obtained the copies from the main campus library and dispensed them immediately to the students. In response to the question to the graduates as to how the college facilitated their degree attainment, 56 percent (87) students commented on the provision for making library materials available as meaningful. The percentage ranged from 41 percent in HSA VII program to 69 percent in the Western Michigan program.

Clinical Sites

Health care agencies in the region were most receptive to having graduate students in their facilities for practice even though previously most had been field placements only for undergraduate students. A variety in size and type of services offered were available so that appropriate experiences could be provided. In many instances, the students identified clinical placements where they wanted to practice and faculty made arrangements accordingly after evaluating the facility. Because of the remoteness of some agencies, it was not always possible to find master's prepared nurses on their staff. However, students were supported by the directors in developing graduate models of practice under the direction of the clinical instructor assigned to the student.

Every effort was made to enable students to practice in agencies close to their place of residence when possible and, in some instances, these were agencies where they were employed. The readiness of these adult learners to gain new experiences, and the acceptance of the directors of these agencies to their staff's student role enabled this role to proceed without difficulty in the place of employment. Since various learning experiences were involved in the program, most students had experience in several settings.

The use of the agencies in the community brought the graduate program closer to those who were in practice and enabled the agencies to benefit from new knowledges which were being explored and developed by the graduate students. Formal contracts with these agencies followed the same procedure as used for on-campus practices sites. Resources in the agency such as libraries, conference rooms, and instructional facilities were readily accessible to faculty and students.

Faculty involved in clinical courses were responsive to questions relative to the quality of the clinical placements. In the first few programs, most faculty felt placements were satisfactory. Several faculty in the HSA VII program expressed some dissatisfaction in placements because of lack of role models, practitioners with graduate preparation in nursing. It was also noted, however, that it was just this lack of graduate prepared nurses that stimulated the college to bring the outreach Master of Science in Nursing program to the region.

Faculty Accommodations

One constant variable in any outreach program is travel; travel by students, travel by faculty and administrators. Travel, housing, meals, and transportation are essential elements in any outreach planning. Although cost factors are discussed in the chapter on costs, certain considerations are addressed here.

Faculty come into an outreach site to work and thus must be assured of quality accommodations. Although cost is a critical factor in pricing any outreach effort, the domain of faculty travel is not an area where budgeting restraints predominate. Facilities where faculty stay must be pleasant with provision for all services faculty need inclusive of exercise facilities such as swimming pools, meal service at any time of day, and other recreational areas to unwind from travel fatigue and concentrated teaching periods.

The type of facilities needed depends on the model by which the program is offered. In the program of the College of Nursing, master teachers in all nursing courses traveled to the outreach site from campus for weekend teaching. On-site clinical instructors came from the region. Some programs use resident individuals as faculty and thus do not need a major budget for housing and meals. Some programs offer concentrated blocks of teaching for a designated period of weeks or months and may prefer other types of accommodations than hotels. In some instances when a program is in an area continuously for an extended time, the sponsoring agency may rent an apartment or purchase a condominium for use by faculty traveling into the site.

In the areas where the College of Nursing program was held, the director of the program negotiated with the manager in a local hotel, inn, or motel for special rates to accommodate faculty. The assurance of continuous reservations over a specified period of several years made the negotiations possible. Rates were agreed on and faculty were assured reservations even in a resort area such as Traverse City where summer is a very busy period. In several instances when accommodations could not be arranged, the outreach office was notified well in advance and the hotel assumed responsibility for obtaining rooms at a neighboring motel for the same agreed on rate. In the early days of the program, budget conditions in Michigan necessitated a decrease in travel allocations. The college accepted the generous offer of space in a dormitory for faculty by one institution and faculty apartments in another. The faculty found these arrangements trying in some ways and felt the need to have more privacy and direct access to meal service. It was this experience that convinced the planners that faculty who take on this assignment need to be "cared for and about."

Per diem rate was the option chosen by faculty in the later programs rather than reimbursement at cost or including meal costs on the hotel bill. Faculty wanted the choice that per diem provided.

Billing is a major concern for faculty, for many find it difficult to handle travel expenses which entail "out-of-pocket" money. Since universities are not known for rapid reimbursement, faculty often had to pay charge card money before the reimbursement arrived. The arrangements in the later programs addressed this concern and eliminated much of the problems associated with outreach teaching. The plan involved cooperation from the hotel and was provided for in the contract. Billing for rooms was sent directly by the hotel billing agent to the outreach office, with faculty paying only for extra personal expenses. The per diem check for each faculty was delivered to the hotel on the morning the faculty was due so that up front money was available immediately for meal expenses. All hotels accepted this procedure and a potential irritant to outreach travel was eliminated. The only billing the faculty person had to submit was for mileage. When air travel was indicated, airplane tickets were purchased directly by the college and given to the faculty member.

Students

Unlike faculty, students must bear their own costs for travel, but the outreach planners do have responsibility for determining accommodations for students who come into the area for classes or other types of experiences. All contracts with hotels provided for the same rate for students as was available for faculty. Arrangements with institutions of higher learning for dormitory space often provided comfortable inexpensive accommodations. Information to students about inexpensive motels and even campgrounds was most helpful. The latter was used frequently in the summer in several programs as students brought their families with them for the weekend.

The economic value of the influx of faculty and students to a region who use the services and facilities in that region cannot be ignored.

Institutions of Higher Learning

In addition to the numerous support services from those institutions already mentioned, the institutions assumed a significant role in carrying out the community-based model. This model was based on the assumption that the College of Nursing would bring only those courses which the community could not provide. The model designated a major role for the local institutions of higher learning to provide the non-nursing courses required in the program.

If a university is available in the immediate region where a program exists, the course offerings are examined and approved when equivalent to course offerings on campus. If a graduate program is not available, the community generally has several universities from the outside who bring graduate programs or courses to the site. This was true in the HSA VII program where the upper part of the lower peninsula area of Michigan has no graduate programs, but other universities such as Northern Michigan University, Michigan State University, and Central Michigan University were readily visible. If any of the courses they brought to the region were acceptable, students were so notified. If not, then one of the universities would be requested to bring in a particular course for the outreach students, but also opened to other students in accord with that university's policy. Only when none of these options were available would Wayne State University offer a course in the cognate area.

This system had many positive benefits and generally facilitated the relationship of the College of Nursing with the community. Student hours were generated for these institutions in the local area and recognition of the value of their course offerings was noted. This provision also provided more choices and flexibility for the outreach students except when a particular course had to be negotiated and brought into the area. In HSA VII where no graduate program existed, the academic dean at North Western College held meetings several times a term with the region representatives of universities supplying courses in the area. The director of the outreach program was invited to be a member of this group as long as the program was in the region.

The representatives discussed their plans for the region and had the opportunity for making requests when specific courses were needed.

The provision for students to earn their non-nursing course credits in local institutions was greatly appreciated by the students. The graduates, 78 percent (120), cited this arrangement as a major means by which the College of Nursing facilitated the attainment of their degree. The percentage ranged from 63 percent in HSA VII to 86 percent in the Western Michigan program. The first program mentioned did not have a university in the region, so it had to rely on those courses which were brought in, while the latter program had a major university in the region, Western Michigan University, which provided for options in the students' program.

Pragmatic issues in this approach are discussed in the chapter dealing with programming. Suffice to say, with the community-based model, use of locally sponsored non-nursing courses could be maximized resulting in decreased cost to the program, satisfaction for the students, and a greater acceptance of the "outsider" institution.

CONCLUSION

Models of programs are visual representations of the organizational structure which serves as a framework for operational decisions. Models based on beliefs about socialization determine the amount of the full program which is actually provided in the outreach location. Models based on organizational structures include satellite centers, partnerships, interinstitutional, or combinations of these.

The community-based model developed by the College of Nursing for its outreach graduate program is a full program model which demonstrates the interrelationship among Wayne State University, the outreach community, outreach clinical facilities, and institutions of higher learning in the outreach region. The program brought to the areas was the full responsibility of the graduate faculty of the College of Nursing. The premise was that the university would bring to the region only those courses or experiences that the community could not provide. The model required much in-kind contribution from the community, clinical agencies, and local educational institutions. Application of the model occurred in the selection of the on-site office, use of instructional resources, book purchasing, use of library resources, clinical practice sites, accommodations for faculty and students, and availability of non-nursing courses.

The community-based model was readily transported into five outreach sites in Michigan with only slight modifications to accommodate to special aspects of a community.

4

Strategies for Organization and Administration

The logistics entailed in bringing a program to an outreach site involve an administration framework which facilitates coordination and the effective and efficient delivery of all components. Such a framework must identify locus of responsibility and decision making for all parts of the enterprise and must reflect the means by which the policies and the procedures of the sponsoring agency are supported.

PURPOSE OF THE ADMINISTRATION MODEL

The program model chosen by the institution for its off-campus program influences the administrative design it develops for delivery of same. Likewise, the type of program affects the design, for special needs may be critical in some programs. Specifically, professional preparation programs have different needs than one finds in general education programs. A constant factor relative to any quality program regardless of model relates to programmatic decisions. The locus of program responsibilities and decisions rests with the appropriate individuals and bodies within the sponsoring institution. That is, the objectives, course requirements, course sequence, and standards for performance and graduation are functions of the college or department offering the program. In the particular outreach program under discussion here, the

43

graduate program in nursing was the responsibility of the graduate·faculty of the College of Nursing.

The administration framework for an outreach program then addresses the *implementation* of the program, not the *development* of the program. There are two dimensions of the implementation aspect:

1. The plan for implementation of the program itself, i.e., schedule of courses, faculty appointments, selection of students, selection of learning experiences which are the prerogative of the on-campus faculty.

2. The actual operations of the plan relative to facilities, resource allocations, support services, etc., which are the responsibility of the person designated to direct the program.

The provision for the planning aspect of the program delivery can be easily incorporated into the ongoing structure of the institution supplying the program whether on a regular or ad hoc basis. It is the framework for operationalizing the plan that is the concern of planners of outreach programs. Certain considerations are important in designing this administration structure. The degree of distance of the program away from the campus raises issues of communication, student–faculty contact, instructional resource availability, record keeping, and financial and other needs of a traveling faculty and student body. Many of these issues require day-to-day decisions and actions; solutions which can be made readily for those programs offered through the satellite model where mechanisms and locus of operations are already in place. However, in other models, an on-site locus of operations needs to be identified with responsibilities and authority clearly specified for the person in charge.

The challenge then is to develop an administration model which integrates both the on-campus and off-campus models so that the program can proceed efficiently and in accord with the policies and procedures of the sponsoring institution. Such a model must enable individuals to function so that the outreach program and its students are not perceived as external to the parent program, but are, indeed, an integral part of the institution's program and student body.

Administration Personnel

Personnel needed to administer such a program are suggested by the framework developed. A general rule of thumb includes the following. The director carries the principle responsibility for the conduct of the entire enterprise. Because administration entails blending programmatic and operational decisions, this individual must be a senior member of the faculty with appropriate rank for the type of program being offered. The director has a home base on campus, but is a frequent traveler to the outreach site. The on-campus staff varies according to size of the student body served, the allocation of operational activities in the office, and the other responsibilities the director has relative to his or her faculty status. An assistant to the director may be in order to handle daily administrative matters since the director may be away from the office at frequent intervals. At least one full-time secretary is essential, with the work load determining any additional needs.

If an on-site office is proposed, a coordinator for that office is needed to direct its multiple daily activities. This individual not only implements the decisions of the faculty, but also makes practical decisions as evidenced by need. A significant role assumed by this person is support to faculty and students and facilitation of student–faculty interaction. This office is an extension of the on-campus office under the direction of the person in charge of the program. A secretary in this office is the other person required to provide secretarial services to the coordinator and to maintain a communication system with a widely dispersed program population.

Variation in personnel is made in accord with the program model chosen for the outreach effort. In instances where a partnership model is in place, the director of the program may also be the coordinator with offices in both locations. The partner to the school is generally in the local area and makes available to the program office space and support secretarial services, similar to the arrangement used by the first program of the College of Nursing. Whatever format is agreed on, it is essential that the administrative staff be sufficient in quality and quantity to move the program in accord with the plan as expeditiously and as efficiently as possible so that the total experience is satisfying and rewarding to students and faculty.

ADMINISTRATION FRAMEWORK FOR
GRADUATE NURSING PROGRAM

The framework developed by the College of Nursing for its outreach program has been based on several important considerations relative to its characteristics. The framework needed to be in accord with the community-based model with faculty control of the program and the community involvement in its implementation. The program brought to each area was a one-time occurrence, thus the administration framework needed to be transferable so it could apply wherever the program was located. The special elements in the graduate program were incorporated in the design. Although there is one graduate program, there are optional clinical nursing specialties that the students could select as majors. Any one of these clinical nursing majors could be brought into the outreach location, thus the design needed to assure that programmatic decisions particular to each major could be maintained within the department where the major is located. In this aspect, graduate programs differ from undergraduate programs where general nursing is the objective to be achieved.

The total process by which students are admitted for graduate study to the university and to the college and the policies and procedures by which students progress through to graduation must be consistent with the on-campus practices and thus monitored and directed through the director of student services in the college. This quality control is represented in the framework.

The administration model of the college for offering its Master of Science in Nursing programs in five sites has met the particular needs of the program in assuring its quality and efficiency of delivery. It is based on providing for a student body numbering from 36 to 80 in distances from 103 miles to 486 miles from the main campus. Figure 3 depicts the administrative model.

The model depicts the dean as the individual ultimately responsible for the total endeavor. The director of the program is directly responsible to the dean, associate dean of graduate studies, and the director of student services. These three senior individuals assume accountability: the associate dean for the quality of the program in accord with faculty and university standards and expectations; the director of student services for adherence to

Figure 3
Administrative Model

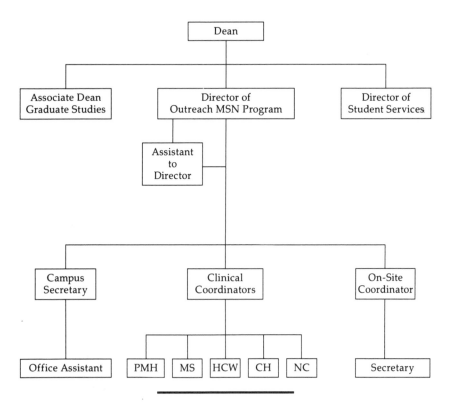

policies and procedures of the college and university relative to graduate students; and the director of the program for the implementation of the program and for its administration in meeting the needs of students and faculty within all budgetary constraints.

An assistant to the director handles many of the administrative details and supervises the on-campus support staff. Two offices are indicated; the on-campus office with a secretary and an assistant to handle the volumes of course materials and communication that are required. The on-site office has a coordinator and a secretary for managing the implementation of the plan in the local area. Both offices are the responsibility of the director.

A different category of personnel appears in this model to accommodate the unique nature of the graduate program. Each clinical department offering a clinical nursing major appoints one of its members to a half-time position to coordinate all activities relating to the students and programs in that field. Five areas noted on the diagram are: MS, advanced medical-surgical nursing; HCW, health care of women; CH, community health nursing; NC, nursing of children; and PMH, psychiatric mental health nursing. The coordinators are accountable to their departments for programmatic issues, and to the director of the program for implementation of the program in the outreach location.

FUNCTIONAL ACTIVITIES

What needs to be coordinated in the administration of such a program? How are these matters coordinated? An examination of the functions of each individual included in the administration framework depicts the multiple activities which must be coordinated in an outreach program.

Dean

Accepts responsibility for the conduct of the outreach program in same manner as for all other programs in the college.

Consults with program director in fiscal matters, resource allocation, and other concerns as indicated.

Approves budget and allocations of monies for the program.

Responds to requests from university administration and other groups for information, etc., regarding the program and its activities.

Attends special meetings in the outreach site; i.e., selected advisory committee, information meetings with students and research day.

Associate dean of graduate studies (Graduate officer of the college)

Assumes responsibility for decisions which affect the quality of the program.

Consults with the director on program matters.

Approves assignment of faculty to teach in the program.

Consults with department chairpersons and faculty on matters of student progression and allocation of traineeship and other scholarship funds.

In accord with on-campus practice, gives final approval for transfer of courses from other institutions; student plans of work which denote the student's plans for meeting the requirements of the degree; outline of the scholarly research project; and graduation credentials.

Attends special meetings in the outreach site as indicated, particularly the student orientation to the program.

Teaches by offering classes or serving as research advisor to students during their independent research project.

Director of student services

Serves as resource person for information relative to university and college policies and procedures for admission, progression, and graduation of students.

Monitors the outreach program in adherence to these policies and procedures.

Consults with director of program and other staff as indicated.

Follows through on actions recommended for students by the college's Graduate Admission, Scholarship, and Promotion Committee.

Arranges for financial aid for students and works with the associate dean of graduate studies in allocation of traineeships and other scholarship assistance.

Evaluates students' records and determines readiness for graduation.

Attends orientation meeting in the outreach site to inform students of graduate policies and procedures.

Director of the outreach program

Assumes responsibility for the implementation of the program directed by the faculty, college, and university.

Develops annual budgets and allocates money in accord with that budget.

Maintains appropriate financial records.

Works with the college administrator and accountant in dispersal of funds and monitoring of the budget.

Determines payment of faculty, staff, and others involved in the program in accord with the college prescribed formula.

Consults with the associate dean of graduate studies, clinical co-ordinators, and faculty on program, course, and teaching matters.

Develops system in office for maintaining student records and monitors its implementation.

Supervises with the associate director the personnel and activities in both offices.

Initiates the operations in the local site; identifies office space, accommodations for faculty, meeting with community leaders, and makes the appointment of the local coordinator and secretary.

Chairs both on-campus and off-campus advisory committees.

Teaches several courses and serves as research advisor to students during their scholarly research project.

Arranges for the teaching of non-nursing courses.

Prepares the annual report.

Serves as consultant to other schools developing outreach programs.

Assistant to the director

Manages all office matters in the absence of the director.

Prepares class schedules for each term.

Assists faculty with preparation of course materials.

Evaluates all transcripts and processes them for admission in consultation with the director of student services.

Evaluates with the clinical coordinator all plans of work and approves with the associate dean of graduate studies students seeking candidacy.

Maintains communication via phone and letter with students regarding their concerns in the program and their progress through the program.

Develops and maintains appropriate record system.

Works closely with the on-site coordinator in operational matters.

Computes cost for each faculty for each term.

Consults with director on plans, issues and other concerns relative to the administration of the program.

On-site coordinator

Develops and maintains a management system in the office.

Consults with the director and assistant to the director as needed.

Carries out duties of the registrar for outreach students each term.

Forwards application data to on-campus office.

Arranges for travel accommodations of faculty and staff.

Reviews hotel bills and arranges for their payment according to the designated plan.

Arranges for faculty/staff per diem checks and delivers them to the hotel for distribution.

Arranges for meetings in the area and prepares agenda and materials.

Maintains a communication system with all involved in the program.

Provides all needed support services for faculty and students.

Prepares newsletter at periodic intervals.

Orders book purchases and other needed supplies.

Maintains a supportive climate in the office for faculty and students.

Works with local librarians and circulates books and materials as indicated.

Helps students in handling their problems and refers appropriate one to director/faculty advisor.

Is a good, empathetic listener.

Serves as liaison for the college, university, community, students, and agencies.

On-site secretary

Provides usual office support services for coordinator.

Prepares typed material for faculty, students, etc.

Maintains communication system with students, faculty, and others involved.

Clinical coordinators (appointed by chairperson of appropriate department)

Acts on admission of all students to the respective clinical nursing major with the assistant director in the outreach office.

Serves as faculty advisor to students in the clinical nursing major.

Holds conferences with students, individuals and groups.

Selects clinical practice sites for students.

Interviews prospective faculty for clinical supervision of students and arranges for their appointment through the college mechanism.

Approves nonclinical nursing courses for students in the clinical major.

Works with faculty teaching in the area.

Teaches at least two courses in the region annually and serves as research advisor for some students.

Maintains communication system with students in the clinical major and with the outreach office.

Approves student plan of work.

Approves class schedule for each term and assists both office staffs in the preparation of class materials.

Consults with the director and assistant to the director and director of student services on matters relating to student progression.

Senior secretary in on-campus office

Provides support services to the director/assistant to the director, clinical faculty coordinator and faculty teaching courses.

Maintains direct communication with coordinator in the on-site office.

Completes appropriate university forms to cover faculty who are traveling and keeps on-going record of money allocations.

Notifies on-site coordinator of faculty/staff travel plans at the beginning of each term.

Arranges payment of faculty travel costs to and from the main campus, including air travel.

Works with assistant director in maintaining student records and such other records as necessary for the program.

Maintains a system for keeping class rolls, dispersing of grade forms to appropriate faculty, and submitting grades to the records department in the university.

Supervises the workload and work of the typist.

Assists director with any support needed in relation to her work.

Assists with office correspondence.

Serves as liaison between the program and all other departments in the university whose services are essential to the conduct of the program.

Typist

Works under the supervision of senior secretary.

Prepares all course material.

Prepares all reference materials to be duplicated and sent to libraries and the on-site office.

Types letters, memos, and other materials sent from the office.

Assists the senior secretary in whatever tasks are needed.

The listing of the activities of various personnel provides insight into the myriad of activities which must be coordinated in planning an outreach program. Communication systems are crucial in planning for any of the positions on this framework. The usual practice of "stopping by" one's office or the dispensing of memos is not effective for a widely geographically dispersed population. Frequent use of the telephone and correspondence through the mails must be anticipated in any planning and the roles and responsibilities of the administration individuals in this function must be delineated.

The position of the on-site coordinator provides a ready access for students who need to be in contact with a university person. This individual can often resolve issues facing the students, but if not, can forward the concern to the appropriate person(s) on campus. Telephone calls to faculty/staff on campus by students are minimized; an important economic factor for students and an important time factor for faculty. The mechanism whereby students can obtain almost immediate assistance with concerns diminishes the feeling of isolation from the main campus and the accompanying feelings of anxiety and uncertainty.

THE IMPLEMENTATION OF THE
ADMINISTRATION MODEL

Throughout the experience of offering programs in outreach sites, the general administration plan has proven most efficient in the delivery of the program with minimal distress to participants. Refinements have been made in response to special factors in the setting, suggestions from participants or program evaluator, or unsuccessful experience in meeting the demands of the endeavor. The framework became institutionalized so that the last few programs were able to develop and proceed with minimal difficulty.

The organization structure of Wayne State University influenced to some degree the means by which the outreach framework was implemented. The College of Lifelong Learning in the university has, as one of its main functions, the administration of all off-campus programs. Other schools/colleges in the university do not have the procedural mechanisms such as registration or recording of grades so that when they go off campus they articulate with College of Lifelong Learning mechanisms. Students register with this college, but if they are students enrolled in another college/school, for example, nursing, then the registration is automatically transferred to the record in the college where the student is enrolled. The significance of the relationship is demonstrated in other parts of this manuscript. Suffice to say, the expertise of the college offering the program is in the curriculum, selection of students, and faculty and the expertise of the College of Lifelong Learning is in the mechanisms for an effective delivery of the program in the outreach location.

Administration Framework—On Campus

When a request for an outreach program came into the College of Nursing and information meetings or other sources had assured an acceptable instructional resources. The need for a locus of operations where decisio could be made when needed was demonstrated in this program; so that wh the college received its own funding, the model of an outreach program on-sit office with a coordinator and secretarial support services was built into the plan. Some modifications in functions occurred as the planners had more experience with the on-site office model.

Appointment of Staff

Decisions relative to the appointment of staff members for the on-site office were determined by their relationship to the on-campus office and the local situations. Because the coordinator handled student records and represented the university in the community, it was decided that that individual would hold an administrative staff position in the university and must meet the requirements as stated in the position description.

The hiring practice used on campus was adhered to: advertisement of the position in local newspapers and the interview of respondents by the director and, in most situations, her assistant. For each program, a cohort of 10–12 people based on timing of receipt of applications was interviewed in a location provided by a community agency. The plan was to form another cohort if there was not a person in the first cohort who met the criteria. No repeat was needed. Several criteria were considered essential in selecting the appropriate person:

Knowledge of the community, its resources and people, since the individual would be the university liaison in the region.

Managerial skills.

Ability to provide support to faculty and students. This is critical since faculty would be doing considerable travel in addition to teaching. Students would be primarily women with responsibilities entailed in work and family. Stress in handling the new role of student with the above pressures would require that the on-site "empathetic ear" with problem solving skills be available to students at critical points in their experience.

Flexibility in work hours to assist faculty and students especially on Friday evenings.

In the interview, it was emphasized to the applicants that the position was one of implementation of a plan of action, not the development of a plan such as many people were used to as coordinator of local or regional health programs.

One complication in the appointment process did occur because of a university requirement that any new position must be posted within the university system and open to any university staff so qualified. The director did

number of students, it was the Graduate Council of the College tha
recommendation to respond affirmatively to the request. The proje
retained responsibility to determine cost needs and seek necessary

The on-campus office handled the numerous inquiries, arran
formational meetings in the region, accepted applications, and evalu
scripts in terms of admission criteria. The selection of students for
was the responsibility of the department chairperson, clinical coord
associate dean of graduate studies, and the director of student servi
designate. The decision as to what clinical nursing majors would be
the region was determined by the number of acceptable students ava
students per major were deemed sufficient in terms of cost and use
resources.

An ad hoc advisory committee was formed by the graduate
guide the program as it developed. The committee included the dire
program, the assistant to the director, the associate dean of gradua
the director of student services and her designate, and the departm
persons/coordinators. Since the program to be taken in the outrea
was the same as on campus, the committee's decisions primarily ∢
implementation such as the decision regarding the clinical nursing
means of handling applicants who did not meet all the criteria for a
scheduling of classes, courses, determining procedures for addressi
travel needs, and other concerns brought to the attention of the gro

In the early programs, this group met frequently, at least tv
times a term, for the newness of the experience required not only
for proceeding, but also the development of procedures for address
unique to outreach teaching. During the past few programs, meet
seldom necessary after the initial one or two at the beginning of a
because the processes and procedures were in place and the indiv
volved were knowledgeable about their roles and responsibilities.

Administration Framework—On Site

The outreach site provided the administration framework w
instances of the new and uncertain. It was the responsibility of the d
the program to obtain and set up an on-site office as a center for op
izing the program. The charge to the office staff was to implement
sions of the college and university on a term or day-to-day basis.

In the first outreach program, the model which was eventual
for all the other programs was introduced by the Michigan Assoc
Regional Medical Programs which assisted with funding for the extra
costs of the outreach program. Office space, a person designated as a
coordinator, and secretarial services were provided in the headquart
Upper Peninsula Areawide Health Planning Association. The Dean o
at Northern Michigan University and Director of the Nursing Progra
Superior State College assumed a major role in assisting with classi

interview on-campus applicants, but the criterion that they reside in the outreach area negated their readiness to fulfill the position.

An excellent coordinator fulfilled the position in Western Michigan and then established residency in Saginaw so as to hold the same position to the HSA VI program. Well organized, well received by the communities and most supportive of faculty/staff/students, she demonstrated the value of such a position to the effective conduct of an outreach program. The second new appointment for HSA VI program proved less satisfactory since the support qualities, demonstrated early in the program, diminished and the role came to be perceived as an information giver. The loss of an "empathetic ear" diminished the value of the office. Termination of the appointment due to residence change resulted in a new person and the office was returned to its significant role in the lives of the students and faculty. Following an interview session, it was the program evaluator in the region who brought the coordinator behavior issue to the forefront for action. Although a negative experience, the value of this position became even more apparent to all involved and influenced the choice of a person in fulfilling the position in the last program. The current appointment is similar to the first appointment, resulting in an open office, strong communication system, and a warm reception by the many community constituents who interact with the program.

The decision relative to the appointment of a secretary in the on-site office took a different approach. In all programs, the on-site office has been located with some connection to another agency; space is provided, but functions are defined by the needs of the program. Other persons in secretarial positions are generally employed in the setting. The secretary to the program was to be a resident of the community. In consideration of the circumstances, the decision was made for the secretary to be hired by the local agency and the university would buy the services of the person for a designated period of time, i.e., pay the salary and fringe benefits according to that agency's policies.

Several factors influenced this decision. Since the secretary would be in an environment where other individuals were employed, the salary and fringe benefits would be the same in accord with the practices in that community rather than different because of the university's scale. In some instances, the scale was lower than at the university; in other instances, the scale was higher. Another factor related to the potential for immediate replacement of the secretary should the occasion arise when the policies and the procedures of the hiring agency were followed. The potential time lapse would be eliminated if the university posting policies and hiring practices were not followed. This system worked in all programs.

Community Advisory Committee

One important element in any administration framework, particularly in a community-based model, is the provision for the community members to have a participant role in the endeavor. After the first program, the community advisory committee was established in each region with the following purposes:

> Guide and make recommendations relative to the implementation of the program.
>
> Provide support to program and students.
>
> Interpret program to the community and serve a "rumor control" function.
>
> Assist in identifying available students, clinical faculty, and facilities essential for the program.

Membership of the committees consisted of directors of nursing in health care agencies, directors of nursing education programs in the region, and one or more student representatives in addition to the director and assistant director of the program. A legitimate question might be raised regarding the limited representation from the community.

The decision of the college to limit representation has a historical root in that period when the first advisory committee was established. The community was conservative with most education occurring in hospitals and with women, for the most part, in a passive leadership role. It was a time when many of the local institutions of higher learning were competing for federal funds for various programs and the state was entering a period of economic distress. The introduction of a well-funded, predominantly women's graduate program into the community was a new phenomenon to be dealt with. In this light, efforts were made by community groups to gain some control over decisions and the possible disbursement of monies. At one point, the director was told by a representative of a group of institutions whom she should appoint to the community advisory committee, mostly representatives of other educational institutions.

It was apparent that if the outreach program impacted the kind of leadership nursing would need in the future, something more than the program itself was necessary. The nursing leadership in the community needed to experience the sense of power and responsibility that accompanies a funded program. Therefore, the decision was made that the committee would comprise the nursing leadership in the area since it was "their program" and their direct involvement was essential in providing and assisting students and clinical faculty for the program and for interpreting the program to the community.

One further effort was made to influence decisions when the community advisory group was invited to form a nursing advisory group in another community organization with the charge to address future nursing education needs in the region. The first area selected by the group was Wayne State University's Master of Science in Nursing Outreach Program. Although the director of the outreach program applauded the decision for a community group to examine needs and make future projections and plans for nursing education, it was necessary for her to clarify the autonomy of the College of

Nursing program in the region with all decisions regarding the program to be the responsibility of the college/university. Outreach decisions for the program could not reside within any other agencies.

The experience of establishing an active advisory group in a community, particularly one for women with a funded program, exposed all to community political pressures and helped to clarify the significance of determining locus of control of decisions in any administration framework. The all-nurse committee learned to function well in the new endeavor and the local educational institutions were pleased to have the students generated by the program in their cognate courses.

The precedent established in the first program was maintained in all other programs. The reputation the college earned for its quality Master of Science in Nursing Outreach Programs influenced the reception and mode of operation in other sites. The all-nurse committee met the needs of the program most effectively, but that is not to say that in some programs the role of other types of committee representation might be advantageous.

The meetings of the advisory committee were held at regular intervals, once a term, but were prepared to meet more frequently as indicated. Regular reports covered program status, student enrollment, program prototypes, class schedules, and program resource needs. Members discussed their concerns, feedback from students in the program, relevant events occurring in the community, and other matters involving the program. Input from students and members was readily solicited in developing the agenda and group problem solving occurred at meetings in response to concerns of members of the college. The committee served a vital role in "steering" the outreach program in the community. The program evaluator met with the committee members and solicited their assessment of the program in the various communities.

Committee members acknowledged the high quality of the program in their areas and the role it assumed in meeting community-based needs. All stated that they were kept fully informed on how matters progressed throughout the designated time period of the program. Their degree of further involvement varied according to opportunities for contact with students in the program. For some, members of their own staff were participants as students; others were involved in providing for clinical experience for students and thus were able to interact with them during courses.

SIGNIFICANCE OF THE ADMINISTRATION MODEL

The model which combined both on-campus and on-site activities proved workable. It promoted coordination of all activities, defined allocation of accountability for the various actions, and enabled all aspects of the program to be addressed appropriately with minimal dysfunction. Evaluative comments from the participants were most helpful in making modifications as the model was operationalized.

Graduates of the program commented on the significance of the outreach office in the local site when asked the question: What recommendations would you make to those who were planning an outreach effort? A consistent theme in the responses spoke to the need to establish such an office with a contact person immediately available. Several graduates commented on the specific characteristics required of the contact person. "Be careful who is picked as local coordinator—he or she must be able to deal with people who are stretched to the limit." Several spoke to the quality of the on-site staff in general. "Screen on-site staff carefully—it's important to have friendly, helpful persons at the on-site office." "Remember the staff and faculty play an important role in retention and satisfaction of students." Recognition of organization as important was noted by several graduates with over 20 graduates recommending that other persons setting up outreach programs use Wayne State University's model.

Faculty responses to the evaluators' questions regarding suggestions to administrators thinking of implementing such a program highlighted two points: acquire community involvement and do adequate planning before the program starts. In identifying components/characteristics/procedures of the Wayne State University program which the faculty felt should be adapted by other programs, two relevant variables were noted: good planning and administrative support.

CONCLUSION

The logistics entailed in administering a degree program away from the campus demand a well-developed administrative framework to assure coordination between on-campus and on-site activities and the efficient and effective delivery of all components of the program. The framework that is developed is a function of the sponsoring agency's model for off-campus programs and the type of program to be taken to the distant site. The framework is for the implementation of the program, not its development. Personnel accounted for in the framework represent the need to assure quality, to minimize hassles which might occur, and to facilitate the student and faculty's experiences within the program.

The community-based model selected for the Master of Nursing Outreach Program required an administrative framework which assured faculty control of the program and community involvement in its implementation. The establishment of an on-site office with an outreach coordinator closely allied to on-campus outreach office and other structures and groups in the college proved a most effective means of fulfilling the obligations inherent in providing a quality experience for all involved.

5

Faculty: An Important Key to Quality

The faculty who teach in a program are key to its quality. This concept is of particular relevance to those planning for an outreach program, because temptation to disavow its true meaning is reflected when expedient answers are sought for questions of cost, faculty workload, commitments of on-campus faculty, scheduling patterns, and situations within the local region. All decisions relative to faculty for a program should be made in terms of the program offered and the institutional policies and procedures which underlie the decisions. Assurance to outreach students that their program is of the same quality as that offered to on-campus students is very much a function of the process used for selection and appointment of faculty.

Questions must be raised as this critical element in an outreach program is addressed. Who will be responsible for and control the program throughout the total endeavor? This query pertains to such items as whether the continuous implementation and monitoring processes are under the aegis of the same bodies as the on-campus program or whether they are the function of another group. In other words, does the program remain as an integral part of the school's operation or does another group take over the school's program and manage it in a new site? The latter occurs when an outside agency such as a hospital or medical center agrees to meet all costs and provide all resources, faculty and others, for a degree program offered in its facilities. It may also occur in situations where institutions of higher learning have schools or departments designated for the development of extension programs. These groups may offer such a program as nursing in outreach sites, sometimes with little or no involvement of the nursing school in that institution.

The answer to the first question influences the response to subsequent questions. Who will teach courses in the outreach program? What will be the qualifications of these individuals and how will the selection process proceed? These questions are directed toward adherence to the related standards and procedures of the sponsoring institution when faculty are appointed to teach outreach courses.

A question not often raised, but of major significance in any quality control, is: What is the relationship of the outreach faculty member to the on-campus faculty and to those campus bodies responsible for program decisions? This question addresses the "we" and "they" phenomenon wherein the outreach faculty are not perceived by on-campus faculty as "one of us" and the concerns and issues which arise during outreach teaching are not matters in which on-campus faculty are involved. In this event, the outreach faculty are truly outsiders, they have no opportunity to participate in the broader activities of a faculty role where colleagueship occurs in decision making which impacts on the program. The outreach faculty teach courses of the department but are not *of* the department or college. The "we–they" phenomenon is a serious matter, for it often is reflected in the on-campus faculty perception of the students. A faculty perceived as "they" often means their students are not perceived as "our" students.

When outreach faculty are considered as "we," they are either part of the on-campus faculty or their workload plan provides for direct contact with on-campus faculty and includes scheduled participation in departmental and other meetings which are related to their outreach endeavors. All notices of policy or procedural changes, events on campus, minutes of meetings, and other items are sent to those outreach faculty whose primary base of operations is not on campus. Likewise, the "we" approach recognizes outreach students as integral parts of the student body, and care is taken to be sure that they also receive notification of events on campus, changes in policies and procedures affecting them, and opportunities for competing for on-campus scholarships and applying for financial aid, honors, or awards.

PATTERNS OF FACULTY SELECTION

In any program, the curriculum including its development, implementation, outcome, and evaluation is the primary responsibility of the faculty. The role of administration is to facilitate the implementation of the curriculum in accord with faculty decisions. Decisions must be realistic within the resources, constraints, and expectations of the institution offering the program. A general practice to assure fit between dream and reality is the involvement of appropriate persons in administration in the curriculum development process.

Because the curriculum, in large part, is the faculty, decisions about faculty assignments to teach in an outreach program become decisions as to the quality of the program brought to the region. Several patterns for selecting faculty for outreach programs have been developed for different programs.

Total On-Campus Faculty

In this pattern, the total program is taught by on-campus faculty who go to the site for classes and other learning experiences. The teaching assignment may be within load so that the outreach teaching is incorporated in the total teaching responsibility of the faculty member. In any one term, such an individual may be teaching classes both on and off campus or may be functioning solely in the outreach site. Another type of assignment is the overload basis whereby the faculty member teaches in the outreach program over and above normal work load and is paid accordingly.

The primary base of operations is on campus and the teacher usually participates in other activities on campus as is compatible with a faculty position. For any one program, outreach faculty may be one person or include various individuals designated for teaching specific content or courses. Whoever is involved, however, has met qualifications for faculty appointment in the sponsoring institution and is recognized as a member of the on-campus faculty.

Total Off-Campus Faculty

In this pattern, all courses are taught by a person or persons in the local region deemed to fulfill qualifications for appointment. Individuals involved should be selected in accord with the standard policies and procedures used for all academic appointments by the sponsoring institution. Unfortunately, this criterion for appointment has at times been compromised by some institutions of higher learning for expediency or as a matter of practice. Various options for faculty appointment exist within the pattern of total off-campus faculty.

One person may be appointed full time with or without academic rank, although the term *adjunct* may be used in the title. This person is responsible for all teaching regardless of the content to be addressed. When one person is appointed, all functions are carried out from an on-site office and the person may or may not have any direct interrelationship with the on-campus faculty or activities within the school. One of the students in the Master of Science in Nursing Outreach Program commented on her experience in a baccalaureate outreach program where she had the same instructor from the local community for all her nursing courses, an individual residing in the community. The student felt that her exposure to multiple and diverse faculty in her master's program was a most welcome and meaningful experience.

A second option is the employment of multiple individuals in the on-site area whose teaching assignments are specific to content areas or courses. Academic rank is generally not accorded and the participants are considered as part-time faculty. It is expected that all involved meet the qualifications for teaching in the program. Teaching assignment is on an overload basis because the individuals are employed elsewhere in the community such as in institutions of higher learning, business, or health care agencies. There is no deliberate attempt to bring these part-time people together. Often they teach a prescribed course, the outline for which has already been approved as an on-campus course. In this case, contact with the sponsoring agency may be through a coordinator and there is minimal, if any, contact with the department offering the course.

This off-campus faculty pattern is most vulnerable to questions about the quality of the outreach program. The "they" phenomenon can occur in it, and many of the activities of the person in a faculty role are carried out without close association with the on-campus persons or groups most concerned with a particular course or experience. In addition, monitoring may be the responsibility of a coordinator who is not necessarily an academician.

A third option entails appointment of a full-time outreach faculty with appropriate academic rank whose base of operations is in the outreach site. The number of faculty is, of course, dependent on the program needs. The individuals function as a faculty under the direction of a program director, and are responsible for all educational decisions affecting the outreach effort within the context of the policies of the sponsoring institution. This pattern has a potential for falling into the "they" phenomenon where on-campus faculty perceive little responsibility for the outreach endeavor.

Whenever reasonable in terms of travel, a safeguard against this perceived separation is for full-time outreach faculty to have some on-campus responsibilities for committees and other activities which entail interaction with on-campus colleagues. This practice also serves as a form of quality control because off-campus educational decisions are then most likely to be in accord with those being made for the on-campus program. Such planning permits faculty travel within the workload, and costs are remunerated. The frequency of contact with the campus is planned to minimize the time for travel yet maximize the time for meeting the desired objectives. The desired goals can usually be attained by investing one day either bi-monthly or monthly.

Combination of On-Campus and Off-Campus Faculty

In this pattern, faculty selected for the program include individuals selected from both the outreach community and the campus on the basis of the expertise needed and available. The outreach programs model indicates if this pattern is appropriate, consideration being given to the available resources and cost factors. Such a pattern provides a wider variety of expertise for outreach students and, in some instances, the increase in resources enables more options to be offered in the site. Several other outcomes are achieved with this pattern. Faculty from both locations are enriched by the sharing that occurs and the community's image and support for the program are enhanced when local people are invited to participate in the educational process.

In this joint approach, the key factor relative to quality control is the role assumed by the on-campus member. The use of on-campus faculty primarily as visiting lecturers does not suffice to assure quality maintenance of the program delivered to the outreach site.

Some plans allocate main responsibility for teaching to the on-campus faculty with regional individuals participating as teaching assistants or in clinical courses as clinical instructors. A close working relationship between the individuals involved in this type of plan is essential if the integrity of the program is to be maintained. Faculty from campus who teach the course must assume responsibility for the total experience; activities for the community faculty cannot be merely delegated without any supervision or consultation.

Some programs select faculty on the basis of expertise or availability regardless of their location. The combination pattern for faculty assignment was the method of choice for the Master of Science in Nursing Outreach Programs offered by the College of Nursing.

FACULTY SELECTION IN A
COMMUNITY-BASED MODEL

The community-based model developed for this program demanded that faculty be selected from both the campus and community. An early decision by the graduate faculty at the College of Nursing affirmed the faculty's belief that the quality control of programs brought to sites off campus rested with the college body. The faculty agreed that the majority of the teaching of nursing courses would be by on-campus faculty. The general statement was that faculty who taught a course on campus would also teach that course off campus if it were offered. Qualified nurses in the local region would be employed on a part-time basis with the primary responsibility for the laboratory course in health assessment and assisting the campus faculty as clinical instructors for clinical courses.

These decisions required modifications in faculty roles, responsibilities, and expectations. Faculty now would be adding considerable travel to their activities, with the need to remain in the outreach area for varying lengths of time. Teaching would now occur in the students' milieu, not that of the faculty. Detroit's community resources, its health concerns, goals, and expectations were well known; the new communities were an unknown. Teaching would now occur away from direct access to familiar resources including colleagues. Accommodation would need to be made between on-campus responsibilities and these new ones entailed in the off-campus program. Changes in lifestyle, personal and professional, were demanded.

Individuals involved in developing outreach programs know only too well that a critical factor in successful outcomes is the willingness of the faculty to bring their expertise to the outreach site. It also is recognized that faculty reluctance or unwillingness to participate are major barriers to any attempt to offer outreach programs. The success of the outreach programs which the College of Nursing provided in Michigan, therefore, was dependent on the positive response of its faculty. How did this response come about?

It would be naive to say that this practice came about without any difficulty. The resistance occurred primarily during the first program which happened to be the one most remote from the campus, a distance of 486 miles. The resistance was not all due to faculty's concerns about teaching away from campus. Other factors were also operating in the college. For example, there was the relatively sudden administrative decision to respond to the desperate need of the Upper Peninsula nurses when funding became available from the Michigan Association for Medical Regional programs. The opportunity was administratively seized, but it did mean that faculty involvement in the decision was minimal.

The decision itself, however, was not far removed from patterns previously established in the College of Nursing. The practice of College of Nursing faculty in bringing courses to out-state sites is historically documented. The general practice was discontinued when the volume of students coming to the college site for graduate study increased significantly due primarily to the availability of federal traineeships. The current master's outreach program was in essence a move to revive and modify an earlier pattern. When the College of Nursing received an advanced training grant from the Division of Nursing, Department of Health and Human Services for completing the first outreach program and initiating a second program, faculty accepted the effort as a total college endeavor and reaffirmed their position that the program implementation and its quality rested with the graduate faculty.

Several activities were initiated to assure faculty involvement in decisions relative to program implementation and the decisions for future programs in other sites. The on-campus ad hoc committee for the outreach program provided a medium for faculty decisions concerning admission of students to the program, courses and other experiences offered in any semester, the selection process of on-campus and off-campus faculty, and standards by which the program was to be monitored and evaluated in relation to the goals of the graduate program.

At the start of a program in a new site, an informational meeting was offered in the area to introduce the Master of Science in Nursing Program to interested nurses. Presentations by on-campus persons, such as the director of the outreach program, associate dean of graduate studies, director of the office of student services, and department chairpersons or their representatives, provided attendees with the types of information needed to make a decision for such a commitment as a graduate professional program would entail. The clinical nursing department representatives had the opportunity to "sell" the virtues of their respective clinical majors which often became a delightful competitive exercise. Once the student body was selected, these same on-campus individuals returned to meet with the students and begin the process of guiding them through their graduate program.

The director made sure that during implementation the faculty's right to make decisions was respected, and sought approval of the Graduate Council of the College before seeking funding and initiating any activities for subsequent programs in new sites.

During the difficult initiation period, faculty met outreach commitments in accordance with their usual high standards, and facilitated the orderly transition to an on-going program in the college. Faculty who taught in the outreach program found rewards from student enthusiasm which reflected for many students the fact that this was their only chance for obtaining a graduate degree in nursing. These pioneer faculty were most helpful in encouraging other faculty to share in this experience.

PERCEPTIONS OF FACULTY
RELATIVE TO OUTREACH TEACHING

Evaluators of the program paid particular attention to faculty perception of roles and responsibilities in the outreach program. A three-step Delphi technique was used to develop an instrument through which faculty members could express their views on this endeavor. Following the first two programs, faculty addressed their receptivity to the program. At the conclusion of this period, 83 percent of faculty indicated that they felt enthusiasm for the outreach program, a positive change from the 56 percent at the beginning of this endeavor. Faculty described attitudes as favorable, satisfied, proud, and supportive. Only 8 percent felt that they were burned out by the experience. The responding faculty indicated that the student responses, watching students grow, student motivation, and playing a role in meeting a need were the most satisfying aspects of the outreach endeavor. They saw the whole outreach effort as advantageous, acceptable, necessary, and a good idea. They felt that outreach programs were feasible, better than proliferating poor independent programs, and essential for nursing to advance. Respondents agreed that there was no feeling that the program exploited faculty.

Data following each of the other programs found general consistency with the first report except that the enthusiasm was much higher in the beginning of each of the program, 73 percent for HSA VI and 68 percent for HSA VII. The latter entailed a much greater distance to the outreach site. Satisfactions were similar except for those reported for HSA VI in response to the student motivation item. This finding is compatible with other data from that region suggesting that the students were less highly motivated than were other students. The HSA VI program was located nearest of all to the campus and other graduate programs. It may be that the students did not perceive the outreach program as the only real option they had to earn such a degree.

Attributes identified earlier relative to the outreach program continued to be rated highly by faculty. One trend was noted in the faculty comments; the increased sense of relief when the program was over, as reported by 42 percent after the first two programs, 67 percent after the third program, and 87 percent after the fourth program. This finding may be a function of the length of the period (12 years) that the program has been in existence.

Once the program was in place and it was accepted by the faculty as an integral part of the college's academic offerings, faculty accepted the challenge and assured high quality teaching. Even though the program is not easy, faculty acknowledged the value of outreach teaching to individuals, the college, nursing, and to themselves.

NURSING FACULTY INVOLVEMENT IN THE OUTREACH PROGRAM

Selection of On-Campus Faculty

As previously stated, the majority of the teaching responsibilities were assumed by on-campus faculty who traveled to the area from campus. Assignment also followed the pattern used on campus. The master prototype of the total program indicated what faculty were needed for each term. As appropriate to each course, the department chairperson in consultation with the associate dean of graduate studies made the outreach teaching assignment after discussion with the specific faculty involved. This approach provided opportunity for departments to share outreach teaching among its graduate members so that no one faculty taught all outreach courses from that major. This procedure helped to prevent burn out for any one faculty member, but more importantly, it enabled the outreach student to experience teaching from several faculty members. This is a continuing practice for on-campus students aimed toward broadening the students' view of their field. Nonclinical nursing courses were usually the responsibility of the nursing systems department and assignments were made in the same fashion used by the clinical departments.

It is noteworthy that most of the faculty assigned to this teaching were senior faculty already established in their fields. This fact did much to assure students that their outreach program was not second class and taught by the least experienced faculty in the college. It also evidenced the commitment these senior faculty felt to their discipline and their responsibility for sharing their expertise with students wherever students may be. The overall quality of the teaching staff and the recognition by the students that their teachers were also teaching on-campus students did much to alleviate any fears the students and the community might have had about the quality of the program that was offered in the area.

Selection of On-Site Faculty

One of the major responsibilities of the clinical coordinators, those representatives charged with administrative functions of the clinical major in the outreach site, was to identify persons in the community who could assist with clinical instruction. Names of nurses with master's degrees in nursing were submitted to the coordinators by students, members of the advisory committee, or other people. After examination of the vitae and an interview, the coordinator submitted the name of the acceptable person to the appropriate department chairperson. The College of Nursing Appointment, Promotion, and

Tenure Committee acted on the appointment in accord with usual policies and procedures. The director of the program and the dean determined salary once approval for the appointment of the part-time clinical instructor was made based on an established formula.

The salary formula used the hourly rate of $12.50 × the number of students to be supervised × the total number of clinical hours in a term as determined by the number of credits allocated—3 clock hours per week equals 1 credit, 1 credit per term equals 45 clock hours.

Example: Rate = $12.50

Number of students = 4

Number of credits = 2

$12.50 × 4 × 90 = $4,500

The number of on-site clinical faculty for any clinical course depended on the number of students in the course, where they resided since practice occurs in their own region, and the number of students which faculty felt they could supervise at any point in time. Thus, a clinical faculty member might be responsible for from one to eight students.

An additional remuneration of $150–300 was added each term for attendance at weekend classes when the on-campus master teacher was teaching. This arrangement provided for quality control by (1) providing for continuity between the classroom and clinical components of the course, (2) involving the clinical faculty in the teaching as a participant in the discussion, and (3) enabling clinical facility and the course faculty to examine issues and develop plans relative to student performance, clinical placements, and learning experiences.

In several instances, alumnae from the College of Nursing residing in the area were designated as course instructors. One appointment was made at the request of students who desired a particular individual to teach a seminar course. In another instance, an alumna was qualified and available to accept an assistant professor faculty position.

The appointment of on-site persons as clinical faculty proved to be a most effective and efficient practice. Knowledgeable about their community, the resources available, and key individuals in the community, these nurses were most effective in providing entrees for experiences which were most meaningful to the students. Performance as faculty was monitored by the clinical coordinator as well as the master faculty for the course. Student evaluations at the conclusion of each course provided performance data, but students also expressed support of or concern with clinical faculty to the staff in the on-site office and director of the program.

The majority of decisions regarding faculty appointments were most successful. In a few instances, when a problem arose, the coordinator initiated corrective action in consultation with the related department chairperson and the director of the program. Problems related to failure to keep commitments, to be prepared for conferences with students, or to plan for experiences. The

formal institution of the clinical faculty attendance at weekend classes eliminated any further problem with the faculty and, indeed, the commitment of
these faculty was greatly enhanced.

Faculty Appointment for Non-Nursing Courses

The community-based model required that non-nursing courses which
were cognates or electives be taught by the institutions of higher learning in
the region. With this arrangement, the institution offering the course assumed responsibility for the appointment of the faculty and the quality of the
instruction. The primary role of the College of Nursing was to approve the
course for acceptance as transfer credit.

The College of Nursing and Wayne State University became more involved when a required course was not available and a Wayne State University
course needed to be offered in the outreach site. One approach involved
requesting the appropriate department on campus to offer the course in the
region by sending one of its faculty as the instructor. This approach was used
in several instances when a genetics course was needed. Since outreach
teaching was not a common practice in some university departments, this
means of sending faculty to teach was not preferred.

The second method was to find someone in the outreach area qualified to
teach Wayne State University's course. When identified to the coordinator or
director of the program, the individual submitted his or her vitae for review by
the appropriate university department. The College of Nursing received notice
of the approval of the appointment from the department and initiated the hiring
process. For the most part, individuals selected held academic appointments in
the surrounding institutions and were often known to the university department members as colleagues within the state. The part-time appointment
meant that the course taught was one of the regular courses offered on campus
and the faculty member was the responsibility of the department housing the
course. This arrangement was used in one or two instances per site.

In the first program, a specially designed graduate course in clinical
physiology was developed by a scientist in the region who had appointments in
several institutions of higher learning. The course plan provided for lectures,
multimedia modular instruction, and clinical seminars. The individual presented the course plan to the physiology department of the Medical School,
Wayne State University, where on-campus nursing students had their physiology course. The department submitted the course to the appropriate university groups responsible for course approval. The course was approved and
considered comparable in purpose and objectives to the on-campus course
and permission was granted by the department to offer the course in the
Upper Peninsula. The same course was also offered in the second and third
programs. This course is described in an article by Whitten (1978).

During the 10 years that the outreach programs were being offered in
the four sites, a total of 37 different on-campus faculty taught courses in the

various regions. Of this number, 5 faculty taught in all four programs, 7 taught in three programs, and 13 taught in two of the four programs. This number of faculty does not include those who contributed as advisers and faculty of note for selected students during their research activities. Clinical faculty from the outreach region numbered 25, and 4 faculty were appointed to teach Wayne State University non-nursing courses. One of these faculty was Dr. Whitten who taught the graduate physiology course in three sites. In the second and third programs, two additional physiologists were employed for each of the programs as preceptors for conferencing the students in their local area since the master teacher lived in the Upper Peninsula.

Evaluation of Faculty Performance

In all programs, selection and appointment of faculty were deliberative processes, an essential means of quality control. On-going data about faculty performance were obtained by the program evaluator in the students' assessment of experiences within their courses. Faculty also obtained data from their students in the same manner as was used on campus, either by using the standard college form or a form of choice. The evaluator's data remained under the aegis of the evaluation study and were summarized for the annual reports of the project. Individual faculty could request the summary report of their own courses. If a significant problem with a faculty member was evident from the data analysis, the program evaluator notified the program director who in turn discussed the issue with the appropriate department chairperson. Action was initiated at that level. It is important to note that the evaluator's data were not used for other purposes such as faculty promotion, tenure, merit raises, for their only intent was to contribute toward the evaluation of the total outreach endeavor. Any other use of the data would detract from its value to program evaluation. Since faculty have other means for obtaining data from outreach students about their performance, they are free to determine the use of data thus obtained. It is usually performance data from this faculty source that are used for institutional purposes at the discretion of the faculty member.

GRADUATES' PERCEPTION OF OUTREACH FACULTY

Documentation of the graduates' perception of the faculty was obtained in the impact study of 154 graduates. Data analysis from the objective component of the questionnaire indicated that 109 (70 percent) of the 154 respondents acknowledged that faculty support was an important means by which the College of Nursing facilitated their attainment of degrees. Out of 12 possible listed items considered influential in this achievement, faculty support ranked third behind items referring to the weekend pattern of class scheduling and the opportunity to take cognate and elective courses in institutions in the outreach community.

In the essay component of the questionnaire, students volunteered comments about faculty under two different headings: (1) general reaction to the program and (2) advice to anyone planning an outreach program.

General Comments

Generally, faculty were highly regarded by the graduates as evidenced in such expressions as: helpful, concerned, dedicated, motivated, supportive, encouraging, excellent both academically and clinically. Quality of instruction was noted by some students who referred to the high standards faculty set for themselves and the students.

Comments most appreciative of faculty were directed toward the policy of having on-campus faculty come to the outreach site.

> One of the best points—WSU faculty never felt we were second class.

> I appreciated the value of campus instructors coming to us.

> Sending regular faculty who likewise showed a personal interest and gave us a flavor of what WSU was all about.

> Utilized top faculty in teaching. This was an outstanding feature and insured that the education offered was indeed of high quality for which WSU is so respected.

Several graduates referred to specific faculty with whom they had studied with such comments:

> Was fantastic—both with knowledge and support.

> Was a breath of fresh air.

> Provided good career model.

> Especially supportive, taught effectively.

> Inspiration to all of us.

Negative comments were few and tended to reflect an individual's personal experience in a student–teacher relationship.

A few graduates reported less than satisfactory experience with faculty, with comments directed toward a particular individual or group of faculty.

> My advisor never addressed me by name.

> I was told by one faculty member that I probably would not make it based on my NLN scores even though I maintained a satisfactory GPA.

Several graduates in the first two programs made comments relative to their perception of the on-campus faculty response to outreach teaching.

Seemed to reflect resentment at being ones to go out.

Faculty often bitched about their assignments and inconveniences. It was hard for me to show sympathy as I too had to change.

Such comments as these were not evident in any responses from students in the last two programs. The comments in the early programs were reflective of two factors. The element of trust was being examined by the students which made the students hypersensitive to any comments by a faculty member. Fear that faculty would not want to continue and the college would then terminate the program before its stated date did exist. As noted previously, faculty also were under pressure in the earlier program, for the decision to start the outreach program was more administrative than faculty inspired.

One graduate described the significance of on-campus faculty in great detail, particularly in reference to three of her teachers from campus.

There were also great teachers who continue to inspire me today. These faculty helped me reach *beyond myself* to strive for my potentials. These faculty made my graduate education such that I could continue to grow when the program ended. To these three I owe a debt of gratitude. I carry their thoughts inside of me as continuous mentors of my professional and personal growth.

Advice to Those Developing an Outreach Program

Concern about faculty appointment comprised a considerable proportion of suggestions from graduates regarding the development of new outreach programs. Such advice from graduates is most significant because they have distanced enough time from their participation as students in the program to offer a meaningful perception of the program from the context of their new professional lives. Use of on-campus faculty to teach was particularly noted by some who made specific suggestions:

Bring chosen faculty to the area.

Bring on-campus faculty to the off-campus site to assure comparable content to on campus.

Do not send the same faculty for all nursing clinical courses.

Make sure faculty are willing to go into the area.

The graduates approve of the use of on-site individuals for teaching, especially for clinical instruction, but did provide some admonitions:

Be sure clinical instructors are interested in what they do.

Please screen adjunct clinical faculty from the community to be sure expertise, goals, etc., are congruent with rest of faculty.

Take advantage of faculty, etc., in the area.

Certain qualities of faculty who teach in the outreach site were specified: qualified, dedicated, warm, adult, supportive, caring, professional, accountable, committed, and "no game playing." Other suggestions were requests for assuring that faculty selection provide for a variety of models and that faculty agree to be accessible to students via phone or other communication devices. One graduate advises, "Remember, faculty and staff play valuable roles in retention and satisfaction of students."

CONCLUSION

Faculty play a key role in the quality dimension of an outreach program; deliberative control over their selection and appointment is crucial. Outreach faculty must meet the institution's standards and criteria for appointment in use for all regular campus faculty. A direct relationship between outreach faculty and on-campus faculty is essential for maintenance of quality control in programs offered away from the main campus, thus assuring that the decisions which affect the outreach program rest with the appropriate bodies in the institution.

Several patterns for selection of faculty are in use in outreach programs: (1) all faculty are regular on-campus faculty who travel to the outreach site to teach; (2) all faculty are selected from individuals in the region who are qualified to teach; and (3) a combination of both on-campus and off-campus faculty. The decision as to the most appropriate pattern is a function of the institution's original model for outreach planning, the availability of resources, both personnel and financial, and the types of expertise required by a particular program.

The community-based model developed for the College of Nursing outreach program required a pattern whereby the major portion of the teaching of nursing courses was the responsibility of the on-campus faculty, but individuals in the region with preparation of at least a Master of Science in Nursing were invited to participate as clinical instructors. The selection of the latter was in accord with the university and college policies and procedures. Faculty teaching non-nursing courses came from the community whenever possible.

Data from graduates evidenced much satisfaction with the plan for melding the expertise of the faculty from campus and community. In general, faculty and students found the experience mutually rewarding. Faculty were responsive to the high motivation and commitment of students while students appreciated the opportunity to study with professionally established teachers from the campus and the access to clinical experts in their own region. Graduates highly recommend adoption of this combined pattern of faculty selection by any individuals contemplating initiation of an outreach program.

6

Strategies for Delivery of an Outreach Program

Many questions arise concerning the actual delivery of a program to an off-campus site. If the program is currently offered on campus, then the issue of sameness must be addressed. Are the words, *same* and *identical*, interchangeable? The difference in meaning of these two terms was discussed earlier. Identical connotes a literal reproduction of the on-campus program in the outreach site whereas sameness implies that both programs have the same objectives, requirements, and evaluation criteria, but are flexible in the scheduling and use of various methodologies to accommodate factors in each location. What types of changes are possible while still maintaining the integrity of the curriculum? What factors determine the type of program offered and the ultimate design of the schedule?

MAJOR CONSIDERATIONS IN THE DELIVERY
OF AN OUTREACH PROGRAM

Type of Program

Planners for any off-campus program must first decide what programs are to be scheduled in the outreach site. For many, the decision will be relatively easy, a program that exists on campus. Others, however, may decide to develop a new program specifically designed for a target group of individuals even though such a program does not exist on campus.

Ongoing Program

When an ongoing program is brought to the outreach site, it must adhere to the standards under which it is presently operating on campus. These standards are determined by the institution itself and any state or accrediting bodies that grant status to and monitor the program.

Standards relate to acceptance of students for the program in accord with the policies and procedures of the sponsoring institution. Standards relate to all dimensions of the curriculum. Not only must objectives of the program and the expectations of the students' performance be the same for both programs, so too should the courses required for the degree and their standards for completion. When the above situation exists, it should be possible, for any student who so desires, to attend a course in either the campus or off-campus location.

However, offering the same program does not mean that the delivery of both programs must be identical. Variation in class scheduling, methodologies, and assignments may be accommodated, although the primary evaluation protocol for each course must be maintained. These modifications are discussed later, but any modification must be in concert with the original intent and must maintain the integrity and quality of the curriculum.

Specially Designed Program

Discussion of this type of program in the outreach area at this point is a recognition of its existence within educational practices in this country but not necessarily an endorsement of such an endeavor. It is not a sound practice for an institution of higher learning to offer a degree program off campus which has no base on campus where control exists relative to program development, faculty approval, and administrative decisions and practices. There may be an instance where the institution's intent is to have such a program on campus but it has already designed the program for offering in the off-campus site in response to a perceived immediate need. This decision is subject to question by educators concerned about quality standards. The complexities of bringing programs off campus preclude the sound introduction of a new program which has not been developed and tested by the campus groups responsible for such actions. Outreach sites are not appropriate locations for such development. Some institutions do offer programs in outreach sites, often far distant from the main campus, which are solely for outreach students and are unrelated to the types of programs generally offered by that institution. Often developed as a means for increasing student enrollment, these programs usually reflect misguided and uninformed notions of appropriate preparation for the targeted group. Since there is no comparable program on campus, the control is housed in some type of extension office. It is in that office that the curriculum is basically developed and packaged for delivery.

Nurses frequently have been compromised target groups for such programs. With blanket credit often awarded for lower level nursing courses taken in a hospital school of nursing or a community college and experience in practice, the nurse is provided with some general education courses from the sponsor, taught not by its own faculty, but by local individuals who are employed on a part-time basis. The degree awarded is a bachelor of health or similar title and has no relationship to baccalaureate preparation appropriate for professional nursing. The message conveyed to this target is that the possession of a baccalaureate degree of some type is the goal without reference to the type of knowledge and skills demanded in practice.

Such programs obviously do not meet the criteria associated with quality and accountability and are not the foci of discussions here.

MODIFICATIONS WITHIN QUALITY OUTREACH PROGRAMS

The design of an outreach program accounts for the accepted course sequence, but does enable the planners to accommodate to factors related to the student body, resources, faculty, and the nature of the environment. Two main factors are the travel requirements for those involved and the working pattern of the students.

Travel affects both the students and the faculty. If the outreach site is perceived to be serving a region rather than one local area, then not all students will reside in the same community as the location of the class sessions. Travel affects time when classes are scheduled, that is, amount of time needed to drive to and from classes can influence the time of day selected as well as the frequency and duration of class sessions. With the travel factor, however, are also climatic factors. Regions with severe winters may not permit the usual class schedules when attendees must travel considerable distance to class. Travel also must reckon with modes of transportation to sites. Although the automobile is the general method of travel, planners must be sure that other ways of accessing the area such as train or plane also exist. During severe winter storms, weather conditions may be too threatening for car travel. If the site is more than several hours drive from the main campus, pressure on faculty time may demand a more expeditious way of travel than by automobile. Time considerations then may be necessary to include in scheduling for various modes of travel.

Travel is not the only determinant of course and class schedule. Characteristics of the student body in terms of ongoing employment must be considered, especially in relation to the offering of a full- or part-time program, the number of courses per term, as well as the time of day when class sessions are held. Travel and employment status of students must be considered together for they influence the same components of scheduling, time, duration, and frequency.

Other factors relate to the availability of faculty and space needs. If on-campus faculty are selected, the work load assignment accounts for travel and teaching time whenever it is scheduled to occur, that is, the weekend teaching time is substituted for other days in its weeks. On-site faculty are sought who can accommodate to the schedule as proposed. Availability of classroom space may be a factor especially if in-kind contribution is a part of the model used for the outreach program. It may be necessary to schedule courses when the institution providing space has less demand on its resources.

Master Plan

When all factors influencing the scheduling of a program are examined, a master plan of the total outreach program is developed by the planners and a copy is distributed to the students. This plan indicates the schedule of courses to be offered for each term, thus assuring students that provision has been made for the completion of required courses. This action is essential for students' planning and for addressing the trust factor, because students' anxiety about the sponsor's willingness to see the program through to its completion often prevails in outreach programs. Some anxiety arose in communities where promises had been made, and institutions failed to keep their commitments. It is understood that unforeseen circumstances may arise which necessitate termination of a program. However, in these instances, the cause should be clear to all and not appear as the result of capriciousness or a change in plans of the faculty or sponsoring agency.

The master plan, often referred to as the program prototype, is most helpful in enabling the sponsor to plan for faculty and other resources for the entire duration of the program. It is especially beneficial for students who are employed, for the plan enables them to project adjustments needed as the program progresses and, thus, arrangements can be made early with employers and families.

Without such a plan, students are unable to plan for their education in the context of other demands in their lives. Students are particularly vulnerable to situational changes occurring when institutions decide to forgo certain classes in a term because of other demands or lack of sufficient enrollment in a particular course. In some programs students may not even be assured that a course is offered until the first day of class. It is true that these changes can occur on campus, but campus students have more options for selecting other courses. An off-campus course cancelled, however, may mean an entire term will be spent without any educational experience toward the attainment of the degree. The prototype charges the sponsor to meet the course commitments except in the most unusual circumstances. In such instances, creative approaches by those individuals from the sponsoring institution and the community may be required to assist students in fulfilling degree requirements.

Scheduling Patterns

Just as a prototype of the total outreach program is essential for the outreach student, so too is the pattern by which classes in the various courses will be scheduled. Each sponsoring institution develops its own pattern in accord with the particular population it is serving and the model by which the total program is developed.

When satellite centers are used, the schedule may resemble the weekly one on campus except for more evening and weekend classes to accommodate the adult working student. Weekly patterns may also be in order when programs are beamed into several areas simultaneously from satellites or through telephone conferencing or television programming. Use of such media strategies may require that individuals meet in designated locations for specific periods of time or, as may be the case with television teaching, the students may view the teaching at home. In the latter plan students may come together for several sessions or may have the entire experience on an individual basis including submission of required material to a specified authority.

When the direct teacher contact is selected as the mode and there is need to serve individuals who must travel considerable distances to the class site, other scheduling patterns are in order, with particular emphasis on use of weekend time at less frequent intervals. Classes may occur on Friday evenings and Saturday, all day Saturday and part of Sunday, or all day Saturday and Sunday. The spacing between these sessions may be every other week, every two weeks, every three weeks, once a month, etc. In selecting the pattern, the time allocation needs to be appropriate to the number of credits assigned to the course. An example follows:

Patterns for a 3-credit course over one semester with 1 credit = 1 hour of class per week for a total of 45 hours. The final examination hours may not be included in the 45 hours.

1. $Q \dfrac{\text{2 weeks — 7 sessions per term + 3 additional hours}}{\text{Friday 6–9; Saturday 9–12 = 6 hours}}$

or

Saturday 8–12 — 1–3

2. $Q \dfrac{\text{3 weeks — 5 sessions per term}}{\text{Friday 6–9; Saturday 9–12, 1–4 = 9 hours}}$

3. $Q \dfrac{\text{4 weeks — 4 sessions per term — 3 hours}}{\text{Saturday 9–12, 1–4; Sunday 9–12, 1–4 = 12 hours}}$

Modification of scheduling can be made within the framework presented here, but it is the total number of hours per session that is critical. Generally six hours at one stretch is the longest period of time that faculty and students can engage in a meaningful experience without undue fatigue.

Another model has been used that has the characteristics of a mini course where intense periods of class are held at frequent intervals over a short span of time, that is, a 12-hour pattern every other weekend for a month. In selecting this model, one must be sure that it is in accord with policies of the sponsor regarding short-term courses and that a mature, self-directed student group is selected, for the intense demands on academic skills of comprehension, analysis, and synthesis within this model are remarkable.

There are variations in class scheduling. Selection is determined on the basis of the particular mix of the student body, nature of the subject to be learned and types of learning experiences required, faculty competencies, and environmental factors such as travel, weather, costs, and so on. Variations in scheduling graduate courses may require approval of the graduate school in universities.

Content

The distribution of course content is influenced by the type of schedule within which it is offered as well as its logical sequencing. When content that is offered weekly on campus is to be organized into more intense weekend patterns, content integrity is examined within other contexts such as the intensity of the class sessions with lessened frequency. Some content may lend itself well to the change in class pattern, whereas other content may require periods of contemplation by the student before it can be related to further content.

For example, in a three-weekend pattern, each time the class meets the content for three weeks of class is taught. In the second weekend session, for instance, classes for week 4, 5, and 6, are scheduled to be taught, but class 5 content needs more exploration and study by the student before it can be related to the content of class 6. Because a time interval between the two classes is not provided, modifications are in order. Class 6 content can be deferred to the third weekend session and another area of content can be introduced for class 6 or an entirely different strategy for teaching the content of class 6 may be used which minimizes or alters its dependency on content from class 5.

Any such modification requires a professional judgment which assures that the integrity of the course is being maintained as consistent with its objectives. Planning the content of an outreach course when subject to a very different time frame does not mean it will necessarily be identical to the on-campus plan. The course must be examined within the new time frame and altered in accord with knowledge of the content itself, the learning process, adults' approach to learning, and the energy resources of both the faculty and students. Creativity and knowledge of university or state-wide system of monitoring graduate programs are called on whenever the fit between on-campus and off-campus content organization is incongruent.

Methodology

Not only may some alteration in content organization be necessary to accommodate a move to a more intense, less frequent schedule of classes, so too many alterations in methods may be required. A concentrated weekend pattern cannot be conducted in the same manner as the weekly pattern of the course on campus, particularly if it is a lecture course. Attention span has limitations which need to be recognized in planning classroom activities. Adults, especially those who are also working as well as attending school, need to be involved in the learning process through various means. In concentrated periods of class a variety of methodologies are in order which provide for different types of stimuli. Just as a long session of lecture can become increasingly less beneficial to students, so too can long periods of class discussion or seminar. Faculty sensitivity to cues from student responses to the learning experience in the classroom and readiness to alter the pacing or method of instruction when indicated are essential components in teaching here. A lecture presentation may be interrupted by a brief buzz session where a problem or issue is given to student groups for discussion and feedback to the large group. Such a session may last only 20 minutes, but the change in the activity provides for a different stimulus in the learning experience. Likewise, when the teacher sees the class discussions reaching the point where student input is minimal and fatigue is evident, a change in direction or perhaps a mini lecture could help the students move forward.

Another activity not usually considered under the concept of methodology is important in long class sessions. The milieu of the classroom takes on considerable meaning in this type of class schedule and can be enhanced by having available a coffee pot, hot water for tea, "goodies" to chew on, and other measures in addition to the usual class breaks. Such may help faculty and students to cope with the long session in the classroom as well as with the demands required for continuous intellectual input as the learning experience progresses.

The emphasis here on methodologies as they pertain to direct teacher student contact is a matter of choice. Previously, the use of various media delivery systems was mentioned as an option for outreach programs and the reader is encouraged to review the literature for data relative to these models of teaching. The use of an electronic delivery system must be examined carefully in light of the goals to be achieved. The method can be most effective if content attainment is the intent. However, for those individuals far removed from the main center of learning, such systems may add to the sense of alienation from scholars in their field which they already feel. The experiences of the College of Nursing in using some of these approaches are presented later.

A further warning comes from Grossman (1987) to the effect that the use of such electronics systems for delivery of educational programs may mean that electronically produced courses which will be used do not represent the individual teacher's way of organizing and presenting the material. Grossman sees teachers as, "changing from creators of instruction to managers of resources and students and from speaking for themselves to disseminating someone else's view" (p. 104). Outreach programs are particularly vulnerable to the misuse of these electronically produced courses. Grossman warns that the system can only be used off campus if the campus faculty develop the package in accord with the campus course. He states, "Quality requires that courses offered electronically be considered the same courses

offered conventionally. If the courses for off-campus students are *not* differen-
tiated from the traditional courses, they will be seen by both faculty and
students as equals" (p. 104).

Methodology for on-campus and off-campus courses need not be identical. It must, however, be so designed as to maintain the integrity of the course
and facilitate the learner's attainment of the objectives. In off-campus teaching,
faculty and student creativity is often called on to enable faculty to experience
different ways of teaching the course content. Often such an experience may
ultimately affect how the on-campus course is taught.

DELIVERY PATTERN OF THE
COLLEGE OF NURSING PROGRAM

Description of the Master of Science in Nursing Program

The Master of Science in Nursing Outreach Program was the same as
that offered to on-campus students; that is, the objectives, course sequence,
and performance outcome standards for each course and the total program
were identical.

The master's program in the College of Nursing is four semesters in
length with a range of from 40–48 credits. The allocation of credits is:

Clinical nursing course	17–24
Cognate or related science	6–9
Research	9–12
Minor or elective	8–12

(the minor is teaching, leadership and administration, geronto-
logic nursing, developmentally disabled nursing, or transcultural
nursing)

The clinical nursing tracks offered through this degree are: advanced medical-
surgical nursing, nursing of children, health care of women, nursing in parent-
ing families, community health nursing, adult psychiatric and mental health
nursing, and child and adolescent psychiatric nursing.

Since the program is accredited by the National League for Nursing,
assurances had to be given that the outreach program met the same criteria
and maintained the same accredited status. This latter point had special
meaning to the students in the program, for regional limitations had denied
many of them access to any accredited nursing program. A separate accreditation report of the first three programs was submitted to the National League
for Nursing because they were started after the college had received its last
accreditation. The programs readily received accreditation status. When the
students in the first program were notified of the accreditation, the director
was taken back by the intensity of the student response. She was reminded by

the students that for many of them this was the first accredited degree in nursing that they had ever earned. The director realized that through this program, nurses were brought back into the mainstream of nursing education and were now prepared to provide leadership in their communities. Protection of the accreditation status meant that the students recognized that they had a quality program.

Master Plan

The length of time a program remained in a particular site was influenced by the availability of outside funds and geographical characteristics of the regions. The minimum period for a part-time program was six semesters to accommodate the four semester full-time program planned for campus. One program, HSA VI, was scheduled for two calendar years, the other three extended over three calendar years. The two programs located in the northern part of the state, Upper Peninsula and HSA VII, did not have nursing courses during the winter months because of the heavy snowfalls in those regions. During the winter term, students enrolled in non-nursing courses, cognate and electives, which were offered at local institutions of higher learning.

In developing the master plan it was essential that the provision for completing the outreach program be demonstrated. Students who wished or were required to go at a slower pace could elect to defer some of their non-nursing courses, unless requisite for a particular nursing course, and their final research project until after the program left the area. They were encouraged to take all courses brought to the region by the College of Nursing or Wayne State University, for each course was a one-time offering. Students who did not complete all degree requirements by the end of the program were followed by the on-campus office and were under the direction of the same faculty coordinator they had while the program was in the outreach site. Advisement for the research study was conducted by mail, telephone, computer, and often individual conferences on campus.

The design of the outreach master plan needed to accommodate both part-time and full-time students. Many students sought nursing traineeships which required full-time study, meaning eight semester hours for graduate study as defined by Wayne State University. Each term the college brought to the region two courses, a clinical nursing and a non-clinical nursing course. This represented a part-time program, but students who wished a full-time program could elect to enroll in one of the non-nursing courses in their program which was offered at a local institution. Figure 4 presents a sample of a prototype for a total program.

The master plan as proposed was maintained in all the programs and no classes were cancelled. The sequence for each clinical program within the master plan was developed by the responsible department in accord with provisions made for those courses which all students take. The selection of a clinical track to bring to the outreach site was based on the number of available students, with

Figure 4
Prototype for a Total Program

Wayne State University
College of Nursing

Revised January 14, 1981
PROTOTYPE HSA REGION VI

MAJOR	Winter 1980	Spring 1980	Summer 1980[1]	Fall 1980[2]
Advanced Medical Surgical Nursing	PSL 0749 (2) Clinical Physiology NUR 0554 (2) Assessment: HX & Phys. Exam.	PSL 0749 (4) Clinical Physiology NUR 0554 (2) Assessment: HX & Phys. Exam. (if not taken) Statistics (if not taken) (CMU)	NUR 0710 (3) Theoretical Fdns. of Nursing Practice and NUR 0603 (3) Organization & Change of Health Care Services Statistics (3) if not taken	NUR 712 (2) Adult Clinical Nsg. I and MINOR SEQUENCE NUR 775 (3) Admin. Process in Nursing or NUR 771 (3) Curriculum Theory Development in Nursing Cognate (3)
Community Health Nursing		Epidemiology (CMU) and Statistics (if not taken) (CMU)	NUR 0751 (4) Adv. CHN NUR 0710 (3) Theoretical Fdns. of Nursing Practice and Cognate (if desired)	NUR 752 (2) Fam. NUR 755 (1) Interventions for Community Health Nursing and MINOR SEQUENCE NUR 775 (3) Admin. Process in Nursing or NUR 771 (3) Curriculum Theory Dev. in Nursing and/or Cognate if not taken
Health Care of Women (Maternity)		NUR 0554 (2) Assessment: HX & Phys. Exam. and Statistics (if not taken) (CMU) Embryology (CMU)	NUR 0710 (3) Theoretical Fdns. of Nursing Practice NUR 0554 (2) Assessment: HX & Phys. Exam. and NUR 0603 (3) Organization & Change of Health Care Services Cognate (2 courses)	NUR 721 (3) Nursing of Women and MINOR SEQUENCE NUR 775 (3) Admin. Process in Nursing or NUR 771 (3) Curriculum Theory Dev. in Nursing

MAJOR	Winter 1981	Spring/Summer 1981	Fall 1981
Advanced Medical Surgical	NUR 713 (3) Adult Clin. Nsg. II and RESEARCH SEQUENCE I NUR 701 (3) Research in Nursing (2 sections) and Select One: NUR 796 (1) Research Practicum NUR 798 (1) Field Study NUR 899 (1) Master's Thesis NUR 753 (2) Nsg. Care of Groups of Psych. course in Group Dynamics	NUR 714 (2) Adult Clin. Nsg. III and MINOR SEQUENCE NUR 776 (3) Personnel Dev. NUR 772 (3) Process of Ed. Prog. Plan. Nursing RESEARCH SEQUENCE II (Select one) NUR 796 (1–3) Research Practicum NUR 798 (1–3) Field Study NUR 899 (1–7) Master's Thesis and/or NUR 785 (2) Seminar in Clinical Nursing	NUR 714 (3) Adult Clin. Nsg. III MINOR SEQUENCE NUR 777 (2) Field Practice in Nursing Admin. NUR 773 (2) Field Practice in Clin. Teaching and/or RESEARCH SEQUENCE II (if not taken) NUR 796 (1–3) Research Practicum NUR 798 (1–3) Field Study NUR 899 (1–7) Master's Thesis and/or NUR 785 (2) Seminar in Clin. Nursing (if not taken) and ELECTIVE NUR 749 (2) Human Sexuality or Cognate (if needed)
Community Health Nursing	NUR 753 (2) Nursing Care of Groups NUR 755 (1) Interventions for Comm. Health Nursing and RESEARCH SEQUENCE I* NUR 701 (3) Research in Nursing and Select one: NUR 796 (1) Research Practicum NUR 798 (1) Field Study NUR 899 (1) Master's Thesis Cognate (2–3) if not taken *Roman numeral is not part of title, used for clarity only.	NUR 754 (2) Nursing Care of Communities and MINOR SEQUENCE NUR 776 (3) Personnel Dev. NUR 772 (3) Process of Ed. Prog. Plan. Nursing and/or RESEARCH SEQUENCE II (Select one) NUR 796 (1–3) Research Practicum NUR 798 (1–3) Field Study NUR 899 (1–7) Master's Thesis and/or NUR 651 (2) Organization & Change of Health Care Services (Formerly 603) if not taken and/or NUR 785 (2) Seminar in Clinical Nursing	NUR 756 (3) Change Strategies in Community Health Nursing MINOR SEQUENCE NUR 777 (2) Field Practice in Nursing Admin. NUR 773 (2) Field Practice in Clin. Teaching and/or RESEARCH SEQUENCE II (if not taken) NUR 796 (1–3) Research Practicum NUR 798 (1–3) Field Study NUR 899 (1–7) Master's Thesis and/or NUR 785 (2) Seminar in Clinical Nursing ELECTIVE NUR 749 (2) Human Sexuality

Figure 4 (continued)

MAJOR Health Care of Women (Maternity)	Winter 1981	Spring/Summer 1981	Fall 1981
	NUR 722 (3) Perinatal Nursing and RESEARCH SEQUENCE I NUR 701 (3) Research in Nursing Select One: NUR 796 (1) Research Practicum NUR 798 (1) Field Study NUR 899 (1) Master's Thesis	NUR 723 (4) Adv. Clin. Prac. in Health Care of Women I and MINOR SEQUENCE NUR 776 (3) Personnel Dev. NUR 772 (3) Process in Ed. Prog. Plan. and/or RESEARCH SEQUENCE II (select one) NUR 796 (1-3) Research Practicum NUR 798 (1-3) Field Study NUR 899 (1-7) Master's Thesis and/or NUR 785 (2) Seminar in Clinical Nursing or RESEARCH SEQUENCE I (if not taken) NUR 701 (3) Research in Nursing NUR 798 (1) Field Study	NUR 724 (3) Adv. Clin. Practice in Health Care of Women II and MINOR SEQUENCE NUR 777 (2) Field Practice in Nursing Admin. NUR 773 (2) Field Practice in Clin. Teaching and/or RESEARCH SEQUENCE (if not taken) NUR 796 (1-3) Research Practicum NUR 796 (1-3) Field Study NUR 899 (1-7) Master's Thesis and/or NUR 785 (2) Seminar in Clinical Nursing (if not taken) ELECTIVE NUR 749 (2) Human Sexuality

[1]Quarter system ends Summer 1980
[2]Semester system begins Fall 1980
The University reserves the right to cancel or change the scheduling of any class when it deems such action necessary.

MAJOR	Winter 1980	Spring 1980 (qtr)	Summer 1980 (qtr)	Fall 1980 (sem)
Psychiatric Mental Health Nursing		Statistics (4) Cognate (4)	NUR 0710 (3) Theoretical Fdns. of Nsg. Practice	NUR 760 (6) Adult Psych. Mental Health Nursing NUR 771 (3) Curriculum Theory Dev. in Nursing or NUR 775 (3) Admin. Process in Nursing Cognate (3)

	Winter 1981 (sem)	Spring/Summer 1981 (sem)	Fall 1981 (sem)
Psychiatric Mental Health Nursing	NUR 762 (4) Psych. Mental Health Nsg. with Groups NUR 701 (3) Research in Nsg. Select One: NUR 796 (1) Research Practicum NUR 798 (1) Field Study NUR 899 (1) Master's Thesis Cognate (3)	NUR 763 (3) Psychiatric Mental Health Nsg. with Groups NUR 772 (3) Process of Ed. Prog. Plan. Nsg. or NUR 776 (3) Personnel Development NUR 785 (2) Seminar in Clinical Nursing Select One: NUR 796 (1–3) Research Practicum NUR 798 (1–3) Field Study NUR 899 (1–7) Master's Thesis	NUR 764 (3) Community Mental Health Nsg. NUR 773 (2) Field Practice in Clinical Training or NUR 777 (2) Field Practice in Nursing Admin. NUR 749 (2) Human Sexuality

Note: Semester Program Requirements:
Major 760–6, 762–4, 763–3, 764–3, 710–2, 749–2, 785–2 = 22
Cognates: Group Dynamics, Theories of Personality,
    Developments, etc. = 9
Minor: Teaching or Administration or Electives = 8
Research: Stat 3, 701–3, 798–3, or 899–8 = 9–14
48–53

Full time 8cr; Traineeship min. 10 cr 1 term, 22 cr 2
terms. For course description see C/N Bulletin 1980–81.

ten generally acknowledged as a minimum number both in relation to cost, and demands on faculty. In several instances, a clinical major was maintained with seven or nine students when the need for nurses prepared in those fields was critical for the community. Advanced medical and surgical nursing was offered in all four programs. Community health nursing and health care of women were offered in three of the four programs and nursing of children was not offered although it is in the current program. Psychiatric and mental health nursing was offered in all four programs.

The master plan designated the non-nursing courses which were to be taken by students in accord with the requirements of the clinical major or the degree itself. As noted previously, these courses were often obtained in local institutions of higher learning and when completed by the student required transfer of credits to Wayne State University. Residency requirements for Wayne State University are not specified in terms of a particular location but rather in terms of a specific number of credits, 24 credits at the master level, taught by faculty of the university and declared as university courses. A requirement for a master's degree from the university states that at least half of the credits in the major field and all research project credits must be selected from courses offered by the university. Any other credits beyond that amount may be earned outside the university. If students have already earned a master's degree in another field, credits earned cannot be transferred to this master's program, but when courses are comparable to courses required for a particular nursing program, courses in the master may be waived, but a minimum of 40 credits is required.

When the College of Nursing generates a course for the outreach program from another institution (e.g., physiology, embryology, group process), a general transfer takes place and the students' grades are recorded on the transcript. Students petitioning for transfer of individual courses (e.g., statistics or other electives) follow the usual process of the university; approval to enroll in the course from the coordinator, submission of appropriate forms and transcript with grade for transfer to the record.

The master plan is also used by students to develop a plan of work which projects the courses to be taken each term so that the degree requirements will be met. The plan, which is submitted after 10–18 credits have been earned, is approved by the coordinator and associate dean of graduate studies in the College of Nursing. Candidacy can be declared with this approval. Any changes in the plan of work require official action from the advisor and the appropriate form noting the action is filed in the student's record.

Class Schedule

Because extensive travel was required for both students and faculty, the emphasis for class scheduling was the clustering of time. A weekend model, including Friday evenings and Saturday, prevailed. In the first program most of the students were teachers and since the winter was so long and the distance so far from campus (almost 500 miles) greater use of the summer months for campus courses occurred. Class patterns during the week were developed—Monday P.M., Tuesday A.M., and Wednesday A.M. The Tuesday P.M. provided for library time for students who came into the main city, Marquette. Many did not have direct access to a major university library and thus could avail themselves of the library at Northern Michigan University in Marquette during this time.

By the second program, the weekend pattern became established and continued to predominate. The number of hours and the frequency of class sessions per term depended on the credit allocation for the course. The most common pattern for a 3-credit course was every 3 weekends × 5. The number of class hours in clinical courses depended on the distribution of credits among class and clinical portions of the course. Some 4-credit clinical courses were divided equally, 2 credits for class and 2 credits for clinical. Others had a 1–3 ratio. Only the classroom portion was scheduled for weekend teaching, although some courses did add additional hours for clinical conferences when all students in the major were together. The practice hours and the clinical conference hours were arranged individually with the on-site clinical instructor and students in accord with the practice credit allocation.

Some modifications occurred in the weekend format. In clinical courses where class credit was designated a 1 credit, faculty often scheduled classes for five hours on three weekends distributed over the term. In one course, Process of Program Planning in Nursing, the instructor planned for a workshop format since the emphasis in the course was for groups of three to four students to work together as a faculty group and design a program of instruction. The plan as developed included Friday evenings and all day Saturday × 4 weekends. The pattern readily facilitated group work by providing for a continuous period of time that students could work together. The latter was particularly important since students resided in a variety of communities often at great distance. The model proved so effective that the instructor used the same weekend format when offering the course on campus.

The pattern for the schedule of course classes that was most effective was planned as follows:

1st weekend   all clinical courses

2nd weekend   all non-clinical nursing courses or science courses

3rd weekend   no classes

This pattern had little flexibility once it was set relative to a particular weekend assignment because the non-clinical nursing courses usually included students from the various clinical nursing majors. Factors which interfered with the maintenance of the pattern were the weekends when holidays or term breaks were scheduled or when the shortened summer period had to be accommodated.

One modification in scheduling involved the selection of sites for courses. Clinical courses were located in the city in which the center of operations was located, primarily because numbers of students, ranging from 7–26, represented an adequate class size. Non-clinical nursing courses, however, involved all students in a particular outreach region, group size ranged from 36–64 members. It was necessary to plan for several sections of these courses; different locations were selected on the basis of where a large mass of students resided. This plan minimized travel for students and also and importantly gave the program visibility in several locations in the region. In the Upper Peninsula program classes were held in the major city, Marquette and in Saulte Ste. Marie, 130 miles apart. In the Western Michigan program classes were held in the primary city, Grand Rapids, and in Kalamazoo, 60 miles apart. In each program similar arrangements were made geographically to distribute class offerings.

Non-nursing courses that were generated in local institutions of higher learning by the College of Nursing for outreach students, although opened to other qualified individuals in the community, followed the weekend pattern. When students enrolled in courses that were a regular offering of the local institution, they attended class at the time at which those courses were scheduled.

Participant's Reaction to the Schedule Pattern

Reactions of participants to the type of schedule pattern used in the outreach programs was sought in the questionnaire sent to the graduates and the tools used by the program evaluators. In response to the question, "How has the College of Nursing facilitated your attainment of the degree?" the highest rating went to the item, the *class schedule*. Many noted that the schedule was well suited to a population that worked and had to travel considerable distance to class. Out of 12 listed items, 86 percent (133/154) chose this particular one. In making suggestions to individuals who anticipate planning an outreach program, the key word suggested by graduates was *flexibility* emphasizing, especially, the need of working students with families. The class schedule met this criterion and many suggested that others use the Wayne State University model.

The evaluators sought faculty reaction to the pattern of class schedules. In the first two programs, 23 percent of faculty respondents felt that presenting long classes was a difficulty while another 12 percent noted no difficulty with the pattern. Most saw positive and negative value to weekend teaching. In the third program, no faculty even considered the plan a difficulty but in the fourth program, 38 percent expressed some difficulty. For this latter program, faculty needed to drive about five hours to class which may be a factor in their perception of the long period of time for classes being a difficulty. One faculty member commented to the director about the different perception of teaching time that the schedule provided for her. Recognizing that the time for teaching was the same for on campus as off campus, the concentrated period for class in the outreach gave her a sense of having more time. As a

Figure 5
Class Schedule for a Semester

SEPTEMBER 1980

Sunday	Monday	Tuesday	Wednesday	Thursday	Friday	Saturday
	1 Labor Day Recess Labor Day	2 Classes Begin	3	4	5 NUR712 (1)* 5–8 pm NUR721 (2) 5–8 pm NUR752 (2) 5–8 pm NUR755 (0–2)Arr. NUR760 (6) 5–8 pm **	6 NUR721 (2) 9–12 NUR752 (2) 9–12 NUR755 (0–2)Arr. NUR760 9–11 am
7	8	9	10	11 Rosh Hashana	12 NUR771 (3) 5–8 pm NUR775 (3) 5–8 pm NUR760 (6) 1–4 pm **	13 NUR771 9–12 noon NUR775 9–12 noon NUR760 1–3 pm
14	15	16	17	18	19	20
21	22	23	24	25	26 NUR712 (1)* 5–8 pm NUR721 (2) 5–8 pm 752 (2) 5–8 pm	27 NUR721 (2) 9–12 NUR752 (2) 9–12
28	29	30		**NUR760 (6) Sponsored by College of Nursing Lecture-Discussion = 3 credits Clinical = 3 credits = 9 clock hours per week ar.	NUR755 (0–2)Arr.	NUR755 (0–2)Arr.

*NUR712 (1) Lecture-Discussion
NUR712 (1) Cl. = 3 clock hours per week (arranged)
NUR721 (2) Lecture-Discussion
NUR721 (1) Clin. 3 clock hours per week (arranged)

OCTOBER 1980

Sunday	Monday	Tuesday	Wednesday	Thursday	Friday	Saturday
			1	2 ··	3 NUR771 (3) 5–8 pm NUR775 (3) 5–8 pm NUR760 (6) 1–4 pm	4 NUR771 9–12 noon NUR775 9–12 noon NUR760 1–3 pm
5	6	7	8	9	10	11
12	13	14	15	16	17 NUR712 (1)* 5–8 pm NUR721 (2) 5–8 pm NUR752 (2) 5–8 pm NUR755 (0–2)Arr. NUR760 (6) 5–9 pm ··	18 NUR721 (2) 9–12 NUR752 (2) 9–12 NUR755 (0–2)Arr. NUR760 9–11 am
19	20	21	22	23	24 NUR771 (3) 5–8 pm NUR775 (3) 5–8 pm	25 NUR771 9–12 noon NUR775 9–12 noon
26	27	28	29	30	31	

NOVEMBER 1980

Sunday	Monday	Tuesday	Wednesday	Thursday	Friday	Saturday
						1
2	3	4	5	6	7 NUR712 (1)* 5–8 pm NUR721 (2) 5–8 pm NUR752 (2) 5–8 pm NUR755 (0–2)Arr. NUR760 (6) 5–9 pm ••	8 NUR721 (2) 9–12 NUR752 (2) 9–12 NUR755 (0–2)Arr. NUR760 9–11 am
9	10	11	12	13	14 NUR771 (3) 5–8 pm NUR775 (3) 5–8 pm	15 NUR771 9–12 noon NUR775 9–12 noon
16	17	18	19	20	21 NUR712 (1)* 5–8 pm NUR721 (2) 5–8 pm NUR752 (2) 5–8 pm NUR755 (0–2) Arr. NUR760 (6) 5–8 pm ••	22 NUR721 (2) 9–12 NUR752 (2) 9–12 NUR755 (0–2) Arr. NUR760 9–11 am
23	24	25	26	27	28	29

DECEMBER 1980

Sunday	Monday	Tuesday	Wednesday	Thursday	Friday	Saturday
	1	2	3	4	5 NUR771 (3) 5–8 pm NUR775 (3) 5–8 pm NUR760 (6) 1–4 pm	6 NUR771 9–12 noon NUR775 9–12 noon NUR760 1–3 pm
7	8	9	10	11	12	13
14	15	16	17	18	19 NUR760 (6) 5–8 pm	20 Classes End NUR760 9–11 am
21	22	23	24	25	26	27
28	29	30	31 Term Ends			

result, she could take a more relaxed approach to discussion and the material presented.

For most faculty, once the longer and more intense class period became familiar, they were able to make the adjustment and look at their teaching in a new light. The periodic concentrated time with students over a weekend enabled faculty to assume a significant role in the professional socialization of the students. Already recognized as scholars in their own right, these faculty had a very special interaction with their students, sharing meals, coffee breaks, and other interactions which helped to foster close relationships with students—such relationships often are not possible on campus. Faculty have commented on how well they knew their outreach students and the students themselves have reflected this view.

CONTENT/METHODOLOGY

These two items are presented together because there was no significant modification in content; it is the methods used to teach the content that vary. The same courses were offered on and off campus and thus the content was not altered except to adjust to the time pattern used. Changes in content from one outreach program to another reflected similar changes in the on-campus program resulting from developing knowledge in the field or the increase in faculty expertise.

Some modifications in method were used. The first program, Upper Peninsula, was far removed from campus and thus seemed a logical site for use of teaching methods which decreased the amount of time faculty and students needed to travel. It was felt that if various multimedia systems were successful in this program, they might become a major strategy in future programs.

All courses in the first program provided for some student–faculty inter-action in the classroom, usually in the first class and at one or two class sessions during the term. The physiology course previously described was primarily modular with study guides, slide tapes, films, and readings located in two sites, Northern Michigan University and Lake Superior State College. During each term (the course extended over two terms), three clinical weekend classes were held with all students, the physiologist, and a physician. The self-study approach in the laboratories was not fully satisfying to many students who felt the need for more faculty participation for clarification and exploration of ideas and meanings. In the following two sites where the program was used, a physiologist in each area where modules were located (two in each region, i.e., in Western Michigan, one was in Grand Rapids and the other in Kalamazoo) was employed to meet with students in seminars and individual conferences as needed. The combination of multimedia, direct faculty contact, and clinical sessions produced a more scholarly result for students.

Telephone conferencing was another method used. In a psychiatric nursing course, students met in two different sites, each site equipped with telephone hook up to the campus telephone so that a dialogue between students and the instructor could occur. Preliminary material relevant to the class discussion was sent to the students before the bi-weekly telephone conferences. The instructor met with the students for the first class and then handled assignments through the mail. The epidemiology course was used in a similar fashion except that video tapes and slide-tape presentations other than telephone conferencing were the predominate methods. Similar to the other course, the on-campus instructor met with the students for the first class and assignments were handled through the mail. In the epidemiology course, several lectures were given from an on-site epidemiologist.

By the start of the second program, skill in history-taking and physical assessment was required for most of the clinical nursing tracks. This course was developed on campus as a self-paced modular course according to body systems with preceptors available to evaluate the student at the conclusion of each module. The same format was used in the outreach programs where sets of material were located in each site and local preceptors were hired. Because skill performance was the goal, this format was suitable for all sites.

The use of multimedia as classroom strategies with the intent to decrease the amount of student and faculty contact was not continued after the first program on recommendation of students and faculty. The students wanted the opportunity for direct interaction with the nursing scholar on a face-to-face basis. The faculty coming into the area was an important element in the students' learning and in accord with their perception of graduate study. The fact that outreach students' distance from the campus denied them opportunities for multiple types of faculty–student interactions made it even more important that the faculty come to the area for classes. The whole approach to graduate education was new to the students and because this program was the only chance for many students to obtain a graduate degree in nursing, they became possessive of the program and the way in which it was conducted.

Faculty found that they were uncomfortable with the multimedia approaches used although they did appreciate the decrease in the number of trips required. Some of this discomfort was undoubtedly due to the newness of the teaching methods, but the faculty too sensed the lack of satisfaction in teaching when students were so far away and there was little opportunity to become involved and get to know their students.

As the program moved into new sites, it became increasingly evident that faculty presence in the teaching-learning situation was a method of teaching in itself which had a meaning greater than the mastery of course objectives. The faculty's use of themselves as models reached beyond their role of expert in their area of nursing. They also represented professionals in the field as a whole and thus became socializing agents in the professional development of their students. Therefore, as models, they not only demonstrated professional expertise in their area of nursing, they also influenced the development of their students as professionals. One of the areas of impact of the outreach program to be presented later addresses the professional behavior of graduates. Undoubtedly such behavior was influenced by this modeling method of teaching in concert with the intensity of student–faculty contact as provided in the weekend pattern of class scheduling.

Use of multimedia became an integral part of the teaching-learning situation as supplemental to the instructional design rather than a dominant method. The seminar method frequently associated with graduate education became the prevailing approach. In the fourth program, the use of computers was initiated and a computer with relevant software packages and connected to the main frame of the university computer was located in the outreach office. Students enrolled in a 1-credit computer course in a community college in preparation for using the computer. The latter was used primarily in handling statistical data computation for students' research projects.

CONCLUSION

Once an operational administrative framework is designed and in place, the on-campus program can be delivered to an outreach site. The program will be the same in terms of objectives, course sequence, and standards of performance in both courses and the total program. Modifications in organization of content and scheduling of classes can be made to accommodate the needs of a traveling faculty and student body as well as employed adults with many demands placed on their time and energy.

A key element in this effort is the early development of a master plan which depicts the sequence of course offerings per term during the designated time period needed for completion of the degree requirements. Such a plan enables the individuals involved to plan accordingly and serves as a statement of commitment by the sponsor to the probability and possibility of the attainment of the goals of the endeavor.

The class schedule is influenced by the nature of the objectives to be achieved, the methodologies selected, and the demands of the environment and the characteristics of the individuals involved. Some form of weekend pattern for class schedule works well for the type of student group that attends outreach programs. Methodologies used must be in accord not only with the objectives of a particular course, but also with the objectives of the total program. In professional programs, this means that mastery of the material and expertise in practice is not sufficient. The process of socialization into a profession is an essential ingredient of such programs and must be addressed in selection of methodologies. The development of direct teacher–student interaction in a seminar format is a significant means to foster professional development.

7

Teaching Skills Specific to Graduate Professional Education: Specialized Clinical Practice and Research

Specialized clinical practice and research skills are two components of graduate professional programs that raise significant concerns of educators when outreach proposals are made. Both skills require a small student–faculty ratio and a milieu with suitable resources to enable the student to attain proficiency at the master's level. Clinical practice skill development requires clinical sites where standards of practice are in accord with those established by appropriate regional and national accrediting bodies and where the climate supports innovation and experimentation with new approaches. Research skill development requires a milieu receptive to the use of the research process in exploring phenomena and replete with scholarly and other resources essential for conducting a study. Can the outreach environment provide opportunity for the student to develop these skills? How is the requisite student–faculty interaction, so crucial to the development of these skills, achieved?

CLINICAL COURSES IN THE OUTREACH PROGRAMS

A teaching area unique to professional outreach programs is provision of practice experience for development of clinical competencies. This component of outreach programs raises many questions, especially by those who perceive that practice can only occur in centers documented as "models" according to selected criteria. It is these types of agencies that on-campus faculty use for students and is often perceived to be the *only* kind of setting where quality learning can occur. There is often resistance or hesitancy to use of health care delivery agencies in rural or other like sites. Yet one of the main purposes for bringing a program to the nonurban community is to assist it in improving the quality of health care it provides. Therefore, any outreach program must consider the use of local facilities as practice field. The action not only accords recognition of the value of these agencies in meeting local health care needs, but also affords opportunities for students to facilitate the development of the various health care services.

The faculty's ability to move within new practice environments, to view their potentials from a less rigid set of criteria, and to sense the challenge and excitement in moving from the "tried and true" greatly influences the success of this endeavor. College of Nursing faculty made several significant discoveries as they moved into nonurban regions. As one faculty said of the students in the Upper Peninsular program, "This is where I see nurses nurse." The lack of health care delivery organizations with territorial claims provided a climate where nurses could be creative in developing programs for the community such as nursing clinics. Faculty also discovered that their outreach students had considerable experience in nursing practice prior to their enrollment. Although this may be related to their age when they entered the program, nonetheless they were quite knowledgeable about the whole spectrum of health care delivery and practices in their respective communities. Several faculty members noted that the latter was not a general finding with students on campus, however. Because graduate students are already practicing in their field and hold a license to practice as registered nurses, the selection of clinical experiences were directed more specifically to their needs and future practice goals. Most undergraduate programs are "clinical-site bound" whereby experiences for a designated period of time are in one locale. Graduate students who are seeking in-depth experiences instead of a breadth of experiences select particular clients representing designated health/illness phenomenon and work with the client in a variety of settings: hospital, home, clinic, etc., within a time frame that is amenable to the client's lifestyle and their own demands. The total clinical practice experience occurs within the specified number of hours per credit allocation, but students control, for the most part, how these hours are allocated and used.

The student and the clinical instructor plan the experience and schedule periodic individual and group conferences which address selected clinical practice concerns. The clinical instructor visits periodically with the student in the practice setting, reviews written work which students prepare in relation to their clinical experience, and maintains telephone communication with students as needed. The latter is important since the clinical experience may not necessarily occur within the usual daytime period. The nature of the clinical experience provides greater flexibility for the student and instructor to maximize potential resources of the community. With the recognition that graduate clinical practice experience differs from that of undergraduate, faculty can support students in their selection of patient problems or health care needs which they wish to pursue.

Programs varied in the number of clinical sites they used, dependent on the objectives to be achieved, the types of experiences available, and their accessibility to students. In the programs, students were graciously received in most agencies and efforts were extended to assure that their learning needs were met.

The clinical courses were comprised of the theoretical portion offered in the classroom sessions in the weekend pattern and the clinical practice portion which incorporated not only theoretical aspects, but experiences in evolving own nursing perceptions as a professional practitioner. The teaching staff, master teacher from campus, and the clinical instructors came together with the students for the weekend sessions where synthesis occurred relative to the total course experience. This plan was important in maintaining quality control over the clinical course, for the planning which occurred asserted that all were pursuing the same objectives.

PERCEPTIONS OF THE
CLINICAL COURSE EXPERIENCE

One of the unknowns in developing the Master of Science in Nursing Outreach Program was the ability to provide clinical nursing courses at the graduate level in remote areas of the state. This question was addressed extensively in the evaluation of the outreach programs from faculty, student, and alumni perspective.

Faculty Perspective

The faculty opinion survey provided data to support the teaching of clinical nursing courses in outreach locations. Between 60–70 percent of the faculty felt that the clinical experiences were less structured and more innovative. They did not concur that the experiences were more designed for students' needs and thus provided for greater freedom of learning than occurred for on-campus students. In the Western Michigan program, faculty felt that the clinical situations for students were no better or worse than those found on campus. In the last two programs, faculty expressed some concern about the lack of role models and its impact on the quality of experience. It is this lack, however, that provided justification educationally for bringing the program to the regions. This lack did require that faculty augment the experience with more conferences and other opportunities for exploring role expectations. In addressing this matter, several students suggested that master faculty from the campus might share periodically their clinical expertise in the clinical setting as well as in the classroom. Visits to the clinical settings and conferences with students about their patients and grand rounds were suggestions.

Student Perspective

Data reflecting the students' perception of their experiences in clinical courses were obtained by the evaluators of the program through the tool, Clinical Course Evaluation Survey, which they developed. The tool was distributed to the students at the conclusion of each term when clinical course requirements were met. Data were obtained from students in the last three programs since it was during the Western Michigan program that the formal evaluation protocol was developed. A further factor involved the program being the same for these three regions—since the major curriculum change occurred at the beginning of the Western Michigan program which placed the clinical component as the major rather than the functional component as characterized in the Upper Peninsula program.

Clinical Course Ratings

An optional five-point semantic differential scale (1 = lowest, disfavorable and 5 = highest, favorable) was the framework for listing items relative to course objectives, instructional assignments and materials, supervision, student evaluations, feedback procedures, and general judgments. When in 1980 the Western Michigan program became the first to be evaluated by this scale, data were also obtained from on-campus students enrolled in the equivalent courses to determine if the outreach program clinical courses consistently rated lower than on-campus courses. The same scale was used in the subsequent two programs.

The bi-modal test was used to judge the level of significance of whether or not items were rated higher by one or the other group of students in the first evaluation. Out of seven clinical courses, four were rated by outreach graduates as well or better than campus sections. The test requires that six of the seven courses would have to be rated higher by students in the same setting to be statistically significant. The data analysis suggested that it is possible to offer clinical courses in outreach areas without diminishing their quality.

A bi-modal test was performed comparing the mean value of Region HSA VI with those of the campus and Western Michigan. Results were slightly less positive except for the overall appraisal items where the HSA VI students were slightly higher. Results were, however, marginally acceptable with an overall mean value for semantic differential response of 3.79. Although less than the mean value of Western Michigan (4.11) and campus (3.91), results were considerably above the mean point average (3.0). The mean for the fourth program (3.49) was the lowest of all programs. Several factors were operating that might have influenced the last rating. In this program the relationship between the on-site coordinator and the students deteriorated and communication became restricted. Here the situation created numerous problems particularly in terms of clinical course work which negatively impacted on student perceptions of their experience. As stated earlier, the person in this position plays a critical role as a support for outreach students who do not have direct access to faculty. A further factor might be related to the perception of some rigidity in some clinical majors when one of the clinical major programs permitted a wide range of cognate courses while others required a more circumscribed selection.

Selection of Clinical Settings

Evaluation data sought information as to the satisfaction of students in selecting their clinical placements. The same semantic differential scale in the Clinical Course Evaluation Survey included items addressing this information. The satisfaction level is expressed as the mean rating on a semantic differential scale: 1 = very dissatisfied, 5 = very satisfied. Table 8 illustrates the method of selection of clinical placement and degree of student satisfaction.

Students generally expressed higher levels of satisfaction with the selection of settings on campus than did the outreach students. Findings for the Western Michigan program are reasonable since it was a new experience for the faculty to plan the new clinical program in a remote area. However, the mean is well above the positive-negative midpoint of 3.0 for the 5-point scale. Increasingly, as the outreach program progressed, students assumed a greater role in selecting their own clinical placements; a practice which seemed to be satisfying. Of course, the placement was required to meet the standards as determined by the particular faculty member involved and approved by same. The students' knowledge of clinical agencies in their regions also enabled them to identify agencies most compatible with their own goals and long-term future plans in relation to course objectives.

The evaluation data suggest that clinical courses can be offered in outreach sites with maintenance of their quality. Each area presents its own uniqueness; planners must be informed as to resources, values, and expectations of the communities. Students strongly support the use of local agencies

Table 8
Method for Selection of Clinical Settings

Region	Selected by Student %	Selected by Faculty %	Jointly Selected %	Satisfied with Process
Campus	43	29	28	4.27
Western Michigan	40	30	30	3.97
HSA VI	55	30	15	4.13
HSA VII	59	23	18	4.14

for clinical practice experience and faculty, although somewhat concerned in instances where role models do not exist, have been satisfied with the experiences provided.

Graduate Perspective

In the section of the questionnaire where graduates proposed suggestions for individuals who were planning an outreach program, several references were made to the clinical practice component of the curriculum, including: struggle to achieve similar clinical component as on campus, provide opportunity to observe clinical nurse specialist working, provide more clinical supervision of clinical experience, have faculty assist with clinical site selection, provide flexibility in clinical experience, use local facilities as much as possible, stay close to the clinical emphasis in the program, and preplan with local agencies. The suggestions of the graduates are consistent with their expressed views when they were responding to the evaluation study as students and thus are significant in any planning for a clinically-based outreach program.

RESEARCH EXPERIENCE IN THE OUTREACH PROGRAMS

Concerns regarding the feasibility of teaching research in an outreach program have risen. With its extensive library offerings, numerous research scholars, and inherent values, which reflect the role of research in its mission as a generator of knowledge, the university campus represents a specific research milieu. Outreach sites where programs are offered are practice rather than research oriented and often lack the resources and support systems necessary for the graduate level of teaching.

The graduate program in the College of Nursing includes a sequence of courses related to research skill attainment: a 3-credit course in statistics, a 3-credit course in research methods, and a research activity with a range from 3–8 credits. The latter may be a (1) field study, (2) practicuum, work on some aspect of a faculty research project, and (3) a master's thesis. This research activity requirement was instituted in the graduate program when the major curriculum revision occurred as the Western Michigan program began. Prior to that, an essay was accepted as an alternative, and many students in the Upper Peninsula program elected the essay option, a pattern similar to that found for on-campus students. In this first outreach program, the essay was fostered by some of the faculty who expressed doubt that a research activity requiring faculty–student tutorial relationship, research library, and other support resources could be conducted at such a distance from the campus.

Once a research activity was required in the new program, faculty efforts were directed toward developing methods for teaching this critical element in graduate education in the outreach sites.

Because the program was located in areas where nursing research was either limited or nonexistent—in contrast to that available to on-campus students where a Center for Health Research existed and contact with faculty researchers was available—the college instituted a Research Day in each site at the time the research course started. The program consisted of research reports from on-campus faculty, doctoral students, and graduates of the master's program representing each one of the three types of research activity options available to the students. In the selection of faculty presenters, consideration was given to some involved in the outreach teaching so as to demonstrate this other dimension of the faculty role.

Although the Research Day program was primarily directed toward the students, invitations were extended to the nursing staff in local health care agencies. Response was generally good and this approach to introducing nursing research was an effective means for setting the climate for the students to carry out their own research endeavor. The presentation of various research models was also helpful to students in their selection of the option they wished to pursue.

The protocol for carrying out the research project was the same as for on-campus students. Some students selected a faculty advisor from those who were teaching in the region. All students received a Faculty Interest Guide which listed faculty in accord with research interest(s). Some students selected their research advisor from that list in accord with commonality of interest.

Student–faculty interaction as required in any research study occurred in various ways. Some individual conferences were held when faculty went to the region for regular teaching assignment. If a particular faculty member had several students, occasionally he or she made a special trip to the site for individual conferences. Much transaction occurred through the mail or telephone. In the later programs, when a computer was installed in the outreach office, some students used the system to transmit their materials to their advisors. As progress in the study development continued, some students chose to come to campus for a conference with their advisor. Students seemed to enjoy this option; for many, this was the first experience on "their campus." If students did not complete their research projects by the time the outreach program left the area, they continued to register for the course and work with their faculty advisors through the usual mechanisms of campus visit, telephone, and mail.

Library resources for research were made available through several mechanisms. In the institutions where reserve books for the outreach program were maintained librarians were most helpful in searches and in obtaining needed materials by interlibrary loan. Many of the books and monographs which the College of Nursing had purchased throughout the program were in libraries readily accessible to students. When indicated, faculty or the director of the program arranged for copies of periodicals which were only available in on-campus libraries. Samples of studies by previous students were made available in the outreach office for student reference. The standard protocol for human subjects was followed both in the college and in the agency involved in the student study.

Once the processes and mechanisms for teaching research in an outreach site were first established in the Western Michigan program, uncertainty over teaching this component of the curriculum vanished.

PERCEPTIONS OF THE RESEARCH EXPERIENCE

Student Perceptions

Because of the uncertainties in teaching research in the outreach site, evaluation was particularly addressed to this aspect for all programs. A Research Skills Questionnaire was developed using a Likart 5-option semantic differential scale with 1 being the lowest rating and 5 being the highest. The questionnaire was sent to the students when they completed their research project. It was also sent to the students in the Upper Peninsula program even though only a few selected a research activity. As with the Clinical Course Survey, this questionnaire was also sent to on-campus students in accord with the same criteria at the time the first questionnaires were distributed in the Western Michigan program. The dates when data were collected are:

Upper Peninsula, Western Michigan, and Campus	1980
HSA VI	1982
HSA VII	1985

The purpose for including the campus students in the first cohort was to determine if the outreach program student research skill development was consistently rated lower for the Western Michigan students than for the on-campus students. Table 9 illustrates a comparison of student responses, both on campus and in outreach programs, on the research skills questionnaire.

The Western Michigan students scored higher than on-campus students, reassuring faculty that the teaching of research skills can indeed be achieved in the outreach sites in spite of some of the limitations previously discussed. The lower ratings for the Upper Peninsula students were expected since many did not engage in a research activity. However, the rating of this group, like all the others, was safely above the positive-negative midpoint of 3. On the specific items, the point below 3 was most evident in two skills: developing an instrument and preparing a complete statistical analysis. Competency in these two skills for most students could be more appropriately achieved in experiences beyond the master's program.

Very few students in each program (1–3 per program) selected the master's thesis. This option required more credits and more time than many students could afford. A similar pattern of choice is found on campus also. Evaluation data on the Research Skills Questionnaire relative to the response on the items in terms of the student's choice of a research activity, field study, or practicuum were examined (see Table 10).

Table 9
Comparison of Student Responses from Campus and
Four Outreach Programs on Research Skills Questionnaires

Program Questions	Campus $n = 46$	U.P. $n = 16$	W.M. $n = 40$	HSA VI $n = 37$	HSA VII $n = 28$
1. Prepared to develop research question.	3.73	3.56	4.20	3.60	3.96
2. How to make a literature search.	4.62	4.31	4.75	4.27	4.49
3. How to find already existing data collection instrument.	3.41	3.44	3.64	3.14	3.99
4. Skill to write an instrument to collect data.	2.82	2.62	3.53	2.60	3.99
5. How to draw a proper sample.	3.66	3.50	4.54	3.81	4.39
6. Prepared to complete statistical analysis of typical data collection.	2.23	2.31	3.13	2.64	2.94
7. Write a quality summary report.	3.15	3.19	4.21	2.97	3.74
8. How likely to engage a literature report prior to enacting steps to address a professional problem.	4.45	3.88	4.64	4.51	4.32
9. Likely to engage in research study to solve a professional problem.	3.60	3.38	3.79	4.63	3.75
	3.52	3.36	4.10	3.57	3.88

Table 10
Comparison of Students' Over-all Rating on Research Skills Development Questionnaires in Relation to Selection of Field Study or Practicum

| | Campus | | Western Michigan | | HSA VI | | HSA VII | | Total | |
	F.S. $n=28$	Pract. $n=18$	F.S. $n=11$	Pract. $n=29$	F.S. $n=23$	Pract. $n=14$	F.S. $n=18$	Pract. $n=10$	F.S. $n=80$	Pract. $n=71$
Rating:	3.54	3.50	4.35	3.87	3.70	3.43	4.04	3.72	3.90	3.48

Scale: 1 = very dissatisfying————5 = very satisfying

The overall ranking in all three outreach programs and the on-campus program suggested that practicuum students were slightly less satisfied with their skill development than were students who elected the field study option. The difference may be a function of the nature of the experience itself or more probably, as was suggested by the last two programs, general distance between faculty and students may interfere with the kind of involvement and interaction needed for a practicuum study.

Graduate Perceptions

The alumnae survey noted that 29 percent, 44/153 of the graduates have been or are currently involved in nursing research. Two have received funding from the Division of Nursing, United States Public Health Service. The majority, 21, have received funding from their employing agency. Other sources include specialty health organizations or community groups. Eight graduates are doing research without external funding.

Various comments from graduates about experience with the research component of their program were volunteered in the open-ended questions. The significance of research to nursing was noted frequently with a particular meaning stated in comments such as, "understanding the use of research was one of the greatest areas of growth, value most the ability to relate research to clinical practice." The experience stimulated interest of graduates in research with several declaring that they plan to contribute to the field. One graduate noted that her knowledge of research was useful in obtaining her present position and another stated that her consultation abilities were greatly enhanced by her knowledge of nursing research.

Several graduates expressed negative feelings about their research experience in the program, stressing frustration and a feeling of discouragement from their faculty advisor in the process of preparing their final research reports. One graduate felt that the program oversold research.

Suggestions were made by several graduates about the teaching of the research component: start earlier in the program and provide for research assistantship experience. One graduate suggested a course on publishing and stated, "Faculty could be a tremendous influence on students by encouraging publication of scholarly papers." Several graduates indicated plans to pursue publication of their research and another graduate stated that the research experience enabled her to write a grant. One graduate wondered if she might have benefited from doing her research on campus where she had greater access to a wider library selection.

Evaluation data suggest that research activity on the master's level can occur in an outreach program. Frustrations that some students experience occur within both on-campus and off-campus programs. Faculty need to be sensitive to the extent that support resources are limited in a practice-oriented environment, but can also maximize that type of setting in helping students develop and pursue their research questions. Library and other support systems can be brought to the outreach site so that such scholarly resources are accessible to students.

CONCLUSION

Two components of a graduate practice program which raise concerns for educators include provision for the development of specialized clinical practice and research skills. Careful planning for such experiences requires recognition of not only the limitations but the resources of the outreach program: what the region can provide for a valuable learning experience. Maximizing community potentials and supplementing community deficits so that sophisticated competency development in clinical practice and research skills can occur are the charge to the faculty because student attainment of such skills represents graduate professional behavior. As a result, quality controls throughout the entire educational process are essential and a monitoring system is necessary.

8

Issues in Budgeting an
Outreach Program

How much does an outreach program cost? What is the relationship between the cost of an outreach program and the cost of the same program on campus? How does one budget for an outreach program? The answers to these questions and others are relevant to both the decisions to offer an outreach program and the type of planning involved.

Methodologies for determining costs of any educational program are tenuous; variables are numerous, complex, and multidimensional. The costing process is particularly difficult in graduate education where such factors as research and need for small faculty–student ratio must be accommodated. It is acknowledged that the most expensive programs in any institution of higher learning are those in health-related fields where practice competencies must be attained by learners. This component further complicates the effort to determine costs of such programs. This factor was noted in the 1974 report, *Costs of Education in Health Professions*, prepared for the Institute of Medicine, National Academy of Sciences.

> The complexity of many health professional schools and the interrelationships between teaching, research, and patient care in the educational process make cost determination difficult and controversial. Data are scarce on costs per students and an aggregate costs for institutions in all health professions. (p. 2)

The development of a proposal of a cost methodology for determining the true cost of an outreach graduate professional program is beyond the purview of this report. Issues in budgeting and resource management for such an endeavor and general principles, however, are relevant to the present discussion. It is assumed that the sponsoring institution has a cost framework and budgeting system for like programs on campus, thus the questions are addressed to those elements which are different in an outreach program and the means by which these differences may be accommodated.

It is generally acknowledged that student tuition in any campus program does not cover the cost of the student's education. Thus, institutions of higher learning seek other means to meet the difference including third-party funding by governmental or private sources, investments, and endowments.

In many instances of off-campus programs, however, there is a general operating principle that declares that the program must be cost effective, meaning that the earned tuition must equal all program costs. Such an approach is predicated on the assumption that a minimum number of students will be enrolled per course, which is a realistic expectation if a single course is to be offered. In situations where a total degree program is planned, such a premise is risky, because many factors can interfere with a particular student's educational plan and may require alterations such as discontinuance in the program, lessening the number of credits earned in a term, or a periodic leave from the program. Such individual problems may result in an insufficient number of students at any given time to meet the course costs; a course may be delayed or, at worst, the total program may be discontinued. The latter action raises ethical questions, for should outreach students be more subject to constant threat of disruption or discontinuance of their program once the institution made its commitment than their counterparts on campus?

Budgeting for outreach programs must be realistic, taking into account the anticipated and unforeseeable consequences of offering any educational program. Need for supplementary money may be required consideration in any budgeting process for outreach programs. Sources for such additional funds may be private gifts, supplementary grant support, sharing of facilities and support services, or the addition of a surcharge on student tuition. Whatever plans are devised, the budget must have some flexibility to accommodate the unexpected.

BUDGETARY QUESTIONS

The following questions are appropriate to be raised by anyone planning an outreach program (modified from list by Todd, 1982, p. 11).

What are the mandated activities?

What contracted services will be required?

What capital costs will be needed?

For what activities will the institution be responsible?

What activities can others do?

What activities are particular cost items in an outreach program?

How can the economic base be augmented?

ANALYSIS OF BUDGETARY QUESTIONS IN TERMS OF OUTREACH PROGRAMS

Mandated Activities

Teaching is the primary activity in an outreach endeavor. Research and community service, the other two designated activities associated with institutions of higher learning, especially universities, may occur, but are generally not considered in outreach budgetary planning. Secondary mandated activities include academic counseling and the usual administrative functions: planning, scheduling, record keeping, and evaluation.

Contracted Services

Personnel costs represent the major budgetary items in this category, with faculty the predominating cost item. Faculty costs are generally related to employment policies and procedures used by the sponsoring institution for payment of salaries and benefits.

On-Campus Faculty.   When regular on-campus faculty are employed, one of two systems is generally used. When faculty are used to teach *in-load*, it means that the faculty member's teaching commitment for any term includes an assignment for outreach teaching, whether as a full- or part-time assignment. In some instances, the portion of the salary which is allocated for outreach teaching may be designated as released time and the dollar amount may be charged to another account such as a grant. Financial compensation to the institution for time required for teaching away from campus enables the institution to employ other persons to assist with the teaching demands on campus.

When a faculty member teaches on an *overload* basis, it means that reimbursement for outreach teaching is in excess of the regular salary. Overload payment generally follows the institution's budget formula, based on credit allocation and rank of faculty member. Some formulas provide for an increment to compensate for time needed to travel to and from the outreach site. This item is different from costs of travel itself. In general, fringe benefits are not awarded on this money.

Another classification of on-campus teachers in the outreach site, summer faculty, is used when the outreach program extends during the summer period. Summer faculty contracts are based on an academic rather than a calendar year. Fringe benefits may or may not be provided in accord with the policies of the sponsoring institution for the employment of summer faculty.

On-Site Faculty. Teaching staff appointed within the outreach site serve in either full- or part-time positions. A full-time appointment is generally in accord with the policies and procedures used on campus and salary is allocated accordingly inclusive of fringe benefits. Part-time faculty appointment is the more common mode with the contract for a particular course. The salary formula generally does not include fringe benefits. In professional programs which require clinical practice skills, another category of part-time faculty may be employed, clinical instructor. The payment formula often differs from the formula used for the usual course as it takes into account an hourly rate, the number of hours of supervision required, and the number of students involved. As with other part-time positions, fringe benefits are not provided in the budget planning.

Administrative Staff. The number of such individuals, whether on campus or off campus, is determined by the outreach model used by the sponsor. The salary is a function of that institution's policies in relation to the position category assigned to the individual. Fringe benefits are included. Administrative personnel may or may not include members of the profession for which the students are being prepared. Some administrative positions may be held by faculty.

Support Staff. Secretarial salary and fringe benefits are in accord with on-campus practices. In the outreach site, it may be necessary to consider the salary pattern customary in the community. A salary package offered by the sponsor that is out of line with the usual community standard, whether higher or lower, can create some difficulty for the outreach staff.

Other Considerations. Depending on the design of the program, other contracted personnel may be provided for in the budget. If program evaluation is an integral part of the plan, and the services of an evaluator are desired, then such services must be budgeted. Payment may be on a contract basis to a particular evaluation organization or may be on an individual basis with a certain amount of time purchased. If a faculty member in the sponsoring institution is selected for the task, then the percent of time purchased also includes fringe benefits. Graduate assistants, students, and others may also be contracted in accord with the payment policies of the institution.

Contracted Services

The model of the outreach program signifies the type of contracted services required.

Instruction Facilities.   These services may or may not require exchange of money. Some community institutions provide such services as in-kind contributions while others require some pattern of payment. If in-kind contributions are provided, then there is no charge to the sponsoring institution for the facilities and therefore no need to include the facilities as a budgetary item. In a satellite pattern, such facilities may be provided in the sponsoring institution's own buildings without charge, or the particular college offering the program may be expected to contribute a specified amount of money toward maintenance of facilities.

Library facilities may be offered as in-kind contributions from on-site agencies or a contracted fee may be established for the services of a librarian in the handling of books and other materials on reserve, or for the use of hardware and duplicating services.

Instructional equipment also may be in-kind contribution or may be on a fee for usage basis. It may be prudent for an institution to purchase or rent such equipment if extensive use is anticipated. The budgeting process must include estimates of cost in terms of the various modes of obtaining equipment. Rental or fee for usage entails some form of written agreement.

Office Facilities.   In satellite centers, the office facilities may be freely available to an outreach program, or the college/department offering the program may be expected to pay a designated rental fee. Office facilities may also be made available as in-kind contribution from some individual or agency in the community, or be rented on a contracted basis unless other interinstitutional arrangements are made. Budgeting for office facilities may also require monies for utilities unless stated otherwise in the contract. Safety mechanisms to protect office equipment and records may also need to be considered as budgetary items.

Subcontract.   Some models for outreach programs use a subcontract in providing for selected on-site administrative functions. This mechanism is particularly useful for programs far removed from campus and not associated with satellite centers. The contract usually identifies a fiscal agent who can pay bills in the local region. Budgeted items in a contract are generally a designated salary amount for the fiscal agent and secretary, travel costs in the local region, supplies, phone, postage, and whatever other costs are required in the on-site program. This type of arrangement provides for immediate reimbursement of local agencies or vendors, eliminates the costly process of submitting all bills through the sponsoring institution's payment system, and enables the employment of local people.

Capital Costs

The financial outlay for capital costs is a function of the model for the outreach program which is used by the sponsoring agency and as it reflects the intent of such an endeavor. The degree of relative permanency in the site is a critical factor in determining capital needs. Capital costs should not be a budgetary item in those programs which plan to be in a region for one or two cohorts of students. In programs that are offered in satellite centers, capital costs are a part of the sponsor's overall budgetary planning, not specific to a particular program being offered through the center, unless specific structural alterations are essential for the program. In outreach programs requiring specific practice facilities (e.g., health professions, computer science, etc.) capital costs for alterations could well be charged to a particular program.

When programs are planned for a long-term presence in an outreach site, capital costs would probably be needed either to build an educational center with appropriate space for offices, conferences, library, computer activity, student reading rooms, practice sites, or to restructure space within a building which is purchased. The decision as to what costs ought to be provided for in the budget must take into account the potential usage of such facilities. A single program effort, even though it will be present in the area over a long-term period, should minimize cost of capital investments, for the pay off is limited.

Equipment and Supplies Required

The equipment needed is directly related to the program model proposed. In some instances the money for equipment and furniture for an office may need to be significant budgetary items. Office equipment today requires new types of machinery such as memory typewriters, computers and printers, calculators, and copy machines. Such equipment may be purchased or rented from a local business concern. If the overall plan for outreach programming entails a long-term commitment or a series of programs in different sites, purchase may be a viable option. The actual decision is a function of obtaining the most cost-effective means.

It may be possible to obtain direct community access to some equipment such as computers and copy machines, with some financial arrangement based on usage. Some office furniture may be available as in-kind contribution from a community agency or business firm.

The usual office supplies are a necessary budget item with particular attention to paper supplies. Communication with a student body dispersed over a wide geographic area often far removed from the main campus entails large amounts of written material: including letters, memos, and notices. Paper for duplicating material such as reference articles and course materials is a significant item. Therefore, one can anticipate greater costs for stationary and paper supplies than is usual for on-campus budgets.

Telephone(s) is another major item that is costly since long distance calls involving on- and off-campus staff and faculty as well as the geographically dispersed student groups are the norm. Budget planning involves examination of the most cost-effective means for providing telephone service, a critical communication device in any outreach program. Systems which may be explored include the various telephone services available in the community: WATTS lines or a long distance service owned by an agency where the office is located.

Instructional equipment such as computers and multimedia hardware and software are budgeted for unless access to them is on an in-kind basis or an integral service of a satellite system.

A budgetary item for book purchase is identified here as instructional equipment; libraries in the outreach site frequently do not contain selected professional literature which is essential to the courses offered. This is especially true for graduate programs in professional fields. If outreach planning anticipates a sequential pattern for outreach programs in different sites, books and other instructional materials could be viewed as a mobile library and thus have greater use. When the program moves to new sites, the purchase of books can be limited to only new editions or new references.

Activities for which the Institution is Responsible

It is an essential quality standard in outreach programs that all activities which relate to program integrity be the responsibility of the sponsoring agency. In some instances delegation of some tasks may be made to specific individuals or groups, but the responsibility can not be delegated.

Activities for which the sponsoring institution is responsible encompass all those which pertain to the delivery of a quality program such as selection of students, program planning, scheduling, selection and assignment of teaching staff, monitoring of the quality of each course and the program as it evolves in accord with on-campus practices, and the counseling of students throughout their program.

Maintenance of a communication system involving interplay of staff and faculty both on- and off-campus, students, and community members is an essential activity which keeps all groups informed, minimizes stress, and serves as a vital role in rumor control. As pointed out previously, communication activities are a significant budgetary item.

Arrangements for travel of faculty and staff to and from the outreach region and within the region itself is a vital activity for which the sponsor is accountable. Not only must arrangements be made, but a system for reimbursement for travel costs to appropriate individuals must be developed and maintained so that bills in the local community are paid promptly and out-of-pocket expenses of faculty and staff are kept to a minimum.

Implementation of registration procedures and other policies and procedures as the students progress through the program is the responsibility of the outreach staff. A crucial activity is the maintenance of student academic records throughout the program in accord with the procedures and practices of the sponsoring institution.

Activities Others Can Do

Support services involve activities that often can be carried out most effectively by on-site persons in the region. Courses such as those in general education, cognates and electives, can be provided by accredited institutions in the region and prove to be a most effective cost saving in the total program. An equivalency system whereby similarly labeled courses among various institutions are examined and equated in terms of objectives and content by the sponsoring institution enables outreach staff to avail themselves of the courses in the area and eliminate duplication of effort. The cost of this component of the professional program is then borne by the on-site institution. In most instances, however it is also revenue generating.

One additional word of caution must be stated here. If a course which is required for a particular outreach program is sought from the local institution, there may be instances where the number of outreach students does not equal the number that the institution feels must be available to make the course cost effective. It should not be expected that the local institution contributes to the outreach program at a financial loss. Sometimes the cost difference is met by increasing enrollment with other individuals in the community. If this is not possible, there may be a need for the sponsoring institution to supplement the local institution's budget so as to meet the discrepancy between the amount of money needed to meet the cost of the course and the amount of money generated by student tuition.

Library services and book purchasing activities within the outreach region can be carried out most effectively by individuals or groups in the community.

In professional programs, especially in the health fields, local professional persons can assist in the identification and preparation of clinical practice sites as well as identification of individuals qualified to teach in the program. Such individuals further serve a vital role in introducing the program to the community and in the identification of resources and potential students.

Activities which are Particular
Cost Items in Outreach Programs

On-site staff of an outreach program need a local base of operation under the direction of a designated individual representative of the sponsoring institution. This appointment is particularly needed when a faculty member on campus is selected as coordinator of the program in order to assure the immediate accessibility to the students of a responsible agent in the community. This is also true whether the program emanates from a satellite center or is a single entity in the region.

The staff may be a secretary, an office manager and a secretary, or a member of the faculty and a secretary. The type of staff selected is a function of the outreach model adopted for the program and the geographical distance between the outreach site and the main campus.

This item is an important budgetary item, for in many ways such an appointment decreases other costs, and by virtue of the continuous visibility of a contact person in the community it is an effective means of keeping enrollment in the program at a cost-effective level. Because students have a locus for obtaining answers, expressing concerns, and completing certain procedural activities such as registration, filing applications for scholarships or other funds, and making program alterations, the students are under less stress in dealing with administrative hierarchies and are more inclined to remain in the program. Communication costs, especially to and from the main campus, are greatly decreased since a knowledgeable individual is readily available. Such a person can answer many questions and is able to target the appropriate responder when answers are not readily available.

Travel.   A major extraordinary cost item in any outreach program is the provision for travel funds. Money budgeted in this item provides for:

1. Faculty and staff travel expenses to and from the main campus as well as travel within the outreach area.
2. Expenses for on-site faculty who reside outside the immediate teaching area.
3. On-site staff travel expenses within the total geographical area of the program as well as some trips to campus when indicated.
4. Special meetings in the outreach site necessitating the transportation of groups of individuals for orientation meetings, special conferences, etc.
5. The director of the program or significant others' attendance at regional or national meetings which have significance for the outreach program.

Money allocation includes:

1. Travel itself on a per mile rate or direct cost as for airplane, bus, train, rented car.
2. Meals in accord with the sponsor's policies whether per diem or direct cost.
3. Residence accommodations.
4. Others such as tolls, cab fare, parking, special tips.

This particular budget item may be vulnerable to cost-cutting measures by planners seeking the most economical means for offering the outreach program, thus resulting in the least expensive arrangements being selected. Faculty travel is the major element in this budget item, however. It is wise, therefore, to view the cost from the perspective of its role in minimizing the stress faculty feel when required to travel considerable distances from their usual setting and support systems in order to fulfill teaching activities. In this instance, the "caring about and feeding" of faculty has a remarkable effect on morale in maintaining their support and minimizing health problems. Budget planning must assure that all travel costs for faculty and staff are met, minimal "out-of-pocket" expenses are required, and that the faculty/staff are in comfortable residences or attractive full service accommodations.

Communication.   A geographically dispersed faculty and student body places heavy demands on communication systems and the equipment and materials essential for operations. As previously stated, generous allocation of money must be made for paper, stationary, postage, telephone, and materials for duplication as well as for the use of communication hardware.

Capital Costs.   Unless a program in an outreach site is designated to exist permanently, capital costs should be minimal, if at all in a budget. Some funding may be needed to restructure some buildings in accord with program needs, but in general, most programs use existing facilities within a satellite center or through a contractual or in-kind arrangement within a community agency.

Equipment.   The extraordinary needs for equipment in an outreach are determined by the type of model used in offering the program. Equipment generally falls in the category of office need or instructional need. Some equipment such as computers and word processors often meet both needs. A modem is often included to enable students to access the main computer frame of the sponsoring institution as well as to communicate with on-campus faculty. Specialized equipment may be required for some graduate professional programs relative to either the research or the clinical practice component of the curriculum.

Augmentation of the Economic Base

As noted earlier, outreach programs require the same consistency in financial support as do on-campus programs. Student tuition is generally not sufficient to meet full costs, thus other sources of money may need to be obtained. When funding for outreach programs is sought from outside agencies, it is important to seek assurance that the support is continuous throughout the period during which at least one cohort of students is in the program. It is recognized that the unexpected may arise that interferes with the projected flow of funds, but if the effort is made in good faith, such an occurrence can be handled by the community and all involved.

Programs which plan for a continuous presence in the outreach site may need extra financial support in the initial offering of the program, but will also need to plan for its eventual inclusion in the institution's overall budget.

Long term financial support—at least two to three years—is best accomplished through grant support, whether from special categories of state budgets, federal fund sources, particular interest groups or foundations. Preparation of such grant requests is a deliberative process which accurately and clearly conveys the essential information requested by the funding agency. Funding is generally not available for planning of programs. The development of realistic plans in accord with delineated needs and the evidence of support and commitment from the sponsoring institution and all other parties concerned are the bases used in determining eligibility for outside funds. Funding is generally programmatic and does not provide money to students to meet their costs.

Another source of outside funding is that which occurs in a partnership model. An agency in the community being served, such as a business, hospital, or community service group, forms a partnership with the sponsoring institution of higher learning and assumes financial accountability for certain budgetary items. This arrangement is generally designated for a specific period of time.

Supplementary funds may also be sought from local agencies or interested individuals in the community. Such funding may assist with the cost of special events in the community, may provide some scholarship assistance to students, or, in the matter of in-kind contribution, may contribute significantly to the cost reduction in providing full services to students in the region.

SPECIFIC BUDGET ITEMS

The discussion of specific budget items as presented is relevant to any budgetary planning regardless of the source of funding and the outreach model used. Major budget headings include: personnel, consultation, equipment, supplies, travel, and other.

Personnel

Administrative Staff. Directors of the program, coordinators, and secretaries are included both on campus and in the outreach site. Costs are generally estimated on a calendar year basis and include fringe benefits. In a cost analysis one might also include the value of in-kind services from the sponsor such as deans, student personnel director, and registrar.

Faculty. All participants to the teaching of students in the outreach program are included, full time, part time, and summer personnel when needed. In planning for part-time faculty, it is best to indicate a certain number of Full Time Equivalents (FTEs) rather than identify specific individuals. The designation of FTEs provides flexibility in selecting individuals to teach so that students have experience with various teachers and the faculty have the opportunity to share the outreach teaching. Money so designated can also be used to cover released time of on-campus faculty when appointed to teach a specific outreach course. This allocation may include on-campus as well as on-site individuals. It is, therefore, advisable to include fringe benefits in the initial budget. If the program encompasses summer months, this plan may designate salaries for 12 months or a separate category of summer faculty may be noted.

The number of faculty needed is a function of the number of students enrolled, the characteristic needs of the particular program(s) being offered, and the scheduling pattern of the program.

Other personnel may be included. If an evaluator is to be assigned, then the salary is stated and may or may not be inclusive of fringe benefits. If a fiscal agent is being used in the outreach site, salary without fringe is included unless the position is for full time.

Consultation

This item may or may not be relevant to a program. It ordinarily includes stipulated fees in accordance with institutional policy, and fringe benefits are not usually included. All travel expenses are included in this item and may reflect more than the per diem costs that are part of the customary travel policies for the members of the institution.

Equipment

The true cost of any equipment is stated. Large outlays of money must be justified in terms of usage and the cost effectiveness of purchase over other means of accessing such as rental.

Supplies

Postage, stationary, paper, duplication of materials, telephone, office supplies, office machinery, books, and manuals are all included in this category. The amount of each item ought to reflect costs as nearly as possible, that is, determining telephone costs in accord with the system selected, determining duplication costs using formula in operation on campus.

Travel

Money allocated in this budget item includes transportation, per diem in accord with the sponsor's policies, and full cost of lodging. Travel costs for each course can be determined by calculating the cost for each trip a faculty takes and then multiplying that amount by the number of trips required for the course (see the illustration below).

3-credit course = 45 hours of instruction (semester)

A schedule every third weekend = 9 hours, requiring 5 trips per course

Mileage—165 miles from campus; total of 320 miles

20 cents (a mile) × 320 = $64.00

An additional $4.00 is added to accommodate any needed travel in the outreach site

Meals—per diem rate of $35.00 @ 2 days = $70.00

Accommodation—$50.00 per night

Total cost

Mileage	$ 68.00
Meals	70.00
Accommodation	50.00
Total	$188.00 × 5 = $940.00 for the course

Variations in the computation will address costs for tolls, faculty extended time in the region for student conferences, or different modes of transportation. If an outreach site is vulnerable to weather which impedes car travel at certain times, it may be wise to plan for that occurring; that is, for two out of the five trips, instead of mileage, include price for airplane and parking at the airport.

Travel for other individuals must be calculated according to a similar formula. The director, evaluator, and others will be visiting the area for a designated number of trips per term. Groups of campus persons may come for a specified number of special events in the site. Some on-site faculty who do not reside in the immediate teaching area may need travel reimbursements when going to the teaching site. In programs where practice in clinical agencies is required, money may need to be allocated for on-site faculty to travel to various agencies for supervision of students.

If the faculty and others are expected to attend regional or national meetings which have significance to the outreach efforts, such trips are budgeted and included in the travel category.

Other

Other expenses may be identified as they relate to the outreach model selected by a particular institution or the special demands of a program within an outreach site. Computer time usage by those in the program may be a budget item. If a subcontract is proposed for the outreach site, it may become a separate budget item. If an outreach office site is managed through a subcontract, then that budget item needs to specify monies for personnel, supplies, travel, and equipment as indicated.

FINANCIAL BASIS OF THE
COLLEGE OF NURSING PROGRAM

In 1975, the College of Nursing was able to respond to the desperate pleas of the Upper Peninsula nursing population for a Master of Science in Nursing program because of the financial support from the Michigan Regional Medical Program where the nursing program was seen as compatible with the agency's goals for increasing health manpower. Prior to this offer, it was acknowledged that neither the college nor the university had the resources to embark on such a costly venture. The money provided from the agency supported all travel costs entailed in sending faculty to the site and even paid part of the mileage of students who traveled more than 30 miles to the program which was primarily held in Marquette, Michigan. Office space was made available in the Upper Peninsula Comprehensive Health Planning Association and the services of a secretary and coordinator were provided. Experience with this model laid the foundation for the ultimate development of the on-site offices in future programs with staff and funds accessible through a subcontract to meet local expenses. All instructional costs entailed with teaching facilities were provided by the two major institutions in the region, Northern Michigan University and Lake Superior State College. The directors of the nursing program in each institution assumed a major role in facilitating all educational experiences and in locating and supporting students and staff.

Although at the time it was known that the regional medical programs were going to be phased out as government programs, it was believed that funding would continue via the new Health Service Agency (HSA) being developed. However, during the first outreach year, word was received that HSA money could only be used for planning programs, not supporting those already underway. With the assistance of the staff at Michigan Regional Medical Program, the college prepared a grant proposal to obtain an advanced training grant from the Division of Nursing, Department of Health, Education and Welfare, United States Public Health Service which would begin July 1, 1976 when the other money source would cease. The request was for three years which would enable the college to complete the Upper Peninsula program and also a program for one cohort of students in Western Michigan from where the college had been receiving requests for assistance. The level of the funding request was based on the community-based model which denoted considerable in-kind contribution from the communities where programs were offered.

The grant proposal was approved for funding, but not at the date requested. That year, the federal government changed its fiscal year from July first to October first so that funds were not made available until January 1, 1977.

The university made a deliberate decision to maintain the program in the Upper Peninsula with assistance from the community during this interim period, July 1, 1976–December 31, 1976, since the program was firmly in place. A response to the Western Michigan request was deferred until funding was assured. A surcharge was placed on the students tuition for each credit (approximately $10.00) to help meet the extraordinary costs in sending faculty to the site. Northern Michigan University and Lake Superior State College made faculty housing available on their campus to College of Nursing faculty coming to the area. This was possible during the summer months when many regular faculty were off campus. All support teaching costs were met by these institutions and the newly organized Upper Peninsula Health Service Agency continued to supply secretarial and registrar services. Through the efforts of all, the program was kept viable until adequate outside funding could be made available. After receipt of the funds for the federal grant. The Upper Peninsula program was completed and the Western Michigan program was instituted.

It was the original intent of the planners that once the outreach program was established with the assistance from the Division of Nursing, funds for future programs would be sought from the state Higher Education budget. However during the Western program, a serious recession struck Michigan resulting in the state's inability to accept new programs for funding. Since the College of Nursing had requests to offer the outreach program in other sites, the college sought continuance of advanced training funds from the Division of Nursing now located in the Bureau of Health Professions, Health Resources and Services Administration, United States Department of Health and Human Services (U.S.D.H.H.S.). Throughout the remainder of the outreach offerings, support from the Division of Nursing continued with competing grant proposals being submitted at the appropriate times. In many ways this approach to preparing individuals at the graduate professional level in off-campus sites where the size of the student population for a continuous program was not viable and where resources and prepared faculty were not adequate was considered most cost effective because no money was needed for either planning or capital outlay. All money requested was spent on the operation of the program itself.

Shortly after the Western Michigan program was "firmly" established with adequate support, a recession occurred nation-wide with Michigan particularly hard hit due to massive layoffs in the automobile industry. Federal funding of programs was particularly vulnerable and in both 1978 and 1979 the advanced training grant was threatened and the continuing availability of federal funds was questionable. At issue was the spiraling national health care costs with questions raised about the need for federal support to increase the supply of physicians, nurses, and other health professionals. With university funds from the state budget drastically cut at the same time, resulting in faculty layoffs and a hold placed on any but essential activities, Wayne State University found it impossible to meet the full costs for continuing the program in Western Michigan. Students and the community were notified of this situation.

On each of the two occasions when continuing fundings were anticipated, but their actual dispersal was in question, the director of the program developed worse case budgets for the outreach programs. This action required proposals for delivering the program so as to reduce costs, recognizing that some students might not be able to meet the demands of these changes. Efforts were made to protect the integrity of the program within these changes. Strategies included: closure of the on-site outreach office, thus decreasing the local support to students and faculty and increasing the work load on campus; decreasing the amount of teacher attendance at classes so that trips could be decreased or requiring that students come to campus for some classes. It was recognized that the latter action would mean that some students could not continue for they too were feeling the pressure of the recession and often were the only breadwinner in the family and could not, therefore, afford to take off time from work. During these difficult periods, there was no suggestion that the program would be discontinued in its entirety and that the students involved would no longer be able to complete their degree requirements.

Fortunately, changes at the federal level provided for a continuous flow of money so that the program could continue as planned with all its quality measures intact and new sites could be accommodated. The financial base of the program included advanced training grant money, student tuition, and in-kind contribution from the community and the administrative services of the college and university.

COST ACCOUNTING MODEL

Little information is available in the literature relative to the total cost of graduate programs in nursing. In general there is no standard formula by which costs of nursing education or any other graduate professional education can be both projected and actually determined. Most of the cost studies in nursing education have addressed baccalaureate education and for the most part only the professional component with little if any recognition of the non-nursing component in the total cost. At present, one might say that any estimated costs of graduate education in nursing are only best guesses.

Most models used for such purposes are unique to an institution and have little general value to the examination of costs on a wide scale. Costs of outreach programs at the graduate professional level have no data base for comparison or analysis. Research, clinical practice, and formal instruction are complex and are not readily amenable to real cost data analysis. In outreach programs, the determination of costs are often a function of the model used, especially when one wishes to determine the cost of a program to a particular institution. Discussion thus far has entailed cost factors within the budgeting process and the varied meanings these factors can have in outreach planning.

Models proposed for use in studying cost factors identify three major categories: direct costs, indirect costs, and capital costs. A model for estimating and analyzing the total cost of baccalaureate education was recently developed as a result of a study by Arthur Young in conjunction with U.S.D.H.H.S. and the American Colleges of Nursing. The model is not institution specific and is to be used to identify total national cost of bachelor of science of degree education programs in the United States. Cost components are defined as:

> *Direct cost components:* compensation (salaries, fringe benefits for full-time, part-time faculty, administrators and support staff); consumable supplies and materials, communications, travel, and

noncapital equipment (for general education, supporting courses for nursing majors, didactic nursing courses, and clinical education).

Indirect cost components: overhead. All allocation of costs from functional areas that support instructional activity (academic support, institutional support, operation and maintenance of the plant, and student services).

Capital cost components: Allocated portion to indirect cost categories and instruction from the value of equipment ($6\frac{2}{3}$ percent of reported beginning year value less beginning year value divided by 2); buildings (2 percent of reported year-end value for annual use charge).

The model is designed for baccalaureate nursing education and could be modified for graduate education, particularly if attention is addressed to the research component cost. Kummer, Bednash, and Redman (1987) report several significant findings that could have meaning for those providing outreach baccalaureate programs.

The Average Cost for Generic Students in 1983–1984 was:

Nursing Component	$3,660
Non-nursing Component	1,768
Indirect	2,721
Total	$8,150

(p. 183)

Table 11 illustrates average cost per credit hour per generic student in 1983–1984.

A further significant finding (Kummer, Bednash, & Redman, 1987) is that the estimated total cost to an institution for producing a generic BSN graduate in 1986–1987 was $51,000 in nominal dollars (p. 184). Professional education at any level is an expensive undertaking. When one adds the extraordinary costs in transporting such a program to regions far removed from campus, then

Table 11
Average Cost Per Credit Hour
Per Generic Student 1983–1984

Cost Category	Mean	Median
Direct nursing	$241	$248
Indirect nursing	121	122
Total nursing	363	379
Direct non-nursing	$ 93	$ 79
Indirect non-nursing	90	40
Total non-nursing	143	119

every effort must be made to keep costs within reasonable bounds with adequate outside support so that the cost of the students attending such a program is not beyond their means.

COST STUDIES OF THE COLLEGE OF
NURSING OUTREACH PROGRAM

The program design using the community-based model had cost control built into it since its inception. The aim to bring from the university to the community only that which the community itself could not provide was a deliberate attempt to control costs and assure cost efficiency while providing a quality program comparable to the program on campus.

The use of the model, however, provides some difficulty in determining the actual cost of the total program for the in-kind contributions were so multiple and varied in nature that their true value cannot be readily assessed.

Cost Considerations

During the 12 years that the College of Nursing program was in operation, several factors led to increases in budget allocations. Inflation during that period had a considerable bearing on the various budget items, particularly as they pertained to supplies such as postage, paper, telephone, and books. Equipment purchase, which in the earlier programs was primarily covered by in-kind contribution, increased in the college budget with the need to purchase computers and word processors. In order to maintain the same quality of educational resources for the outreach students as for those on campus, the latter equipment was essential for the students' research activity.

Personnel salary reflected not only inflation, but also a change in educational preparation of faculty. During the 12-year period there was a steady increase in the use of doctorally prepared, research oriented faculty involved in both the on-campus and outreach teaching. These faculty received higher salaries than those of earlier periods based not only on inflation but also in recognition of their preparation and expertise. Differences in the number of personnel required and thus the amount budgeted in each site were related to the number of students in the particular program, the number of clinical programs offered within the area, and the degree and amount of supervision required. It should be noted that the cost of individual faculty not directly involved in the outreach program who served as research advisors to specific outreach students was a College of Nursing expenditure and not included in the figures.

Travel allocation also reflected inflation in fuel costs, public transportation rate increases, and the charge for lodging and per diem. Transportation costs in each region were functions of the distance from the campus, the means of transportation required, and number of persons traveling.

Each budget report represented the demands at the time and the prevalent costs of staff, services, and supplies. If grant money is being used, then the indirect costs associated with the administration of grant funds must be considered.

In any outreach program, direct costs constitute a majority of the budget. In a community-based model where the in-kind contribution from the community constitutes the major part of the indirect cost and is inclusive of instructional support costs which are often associated with the direct cost category, the majority of funds are for direct costs. In that category, personnel costs represent about 68–72 percent of the direct cost budget in the programs which the College of Nursing offered.

Efforts to do a retrospective study of costs for one year of each of the programs in the four major categories—personnel, equipment, supplies, travel —and others were not successful. During the time period that the programs covered, the format of accounting report records in the university changed and items in some categories were altered. One item that could be readily identified was the direct cost of personnel including salary and wages and fringe benefits. Personnel costs did not include the salary paid to the on-site fiscal agent and on-site secretary (salary was included in the subcontract) and the portion of time considered as in-kind contribution for the services of key people in the college and university. The percentage of time that these key people contributed to the outreach program was estimated to be; Dean—8 percent, Associate Dean of Graduate Studies—10 percent, Director of Office of Research and Sponsored Programs—1 percent, Administrative Officer of the College of Nursing—5 percent, Accounting Assistant—5 percent, Assistant to the Dean—3 percent, Computer Consultant—5 percent, Director of Student Services—10 percent, and Director of the Center for Health Research—3 percent.

The personnel costs are influenced by the number of students and the number of clinical nursing majors offered in the site, because specialized faculty are required for each clinical nursing major and the numbers of on-site clinical faculty are related to the number of students that can be supervised. Table 12 illustrates the numbers of students and clinical majors offered in three outreach programs.

Personnel costs for one year of each of the outreach programs were determined. Personnel costs (salary and fringe benefits) consisted of the

Table 12
Number of Students and Clinical Majors
Offered in Three Outreach Programs

	WM	HSA VI	HSA VII
Number of students	65	52	25
Number of clinical nursing majors	4	3	2

Table 13
Personnel Costs for One Year in
Each of Three Outreach Programs

	WM 1/1/77-12/31/77	HSA VI 1/1/81-12/31/81	HSA VII 3/1/83-2/28/84
Salary and wages	$153,499	$162,618	$166,063
Fringe benefits	17,895	21,149	24,846
Total	$171,394	$183,767	$190,909

on-campus administrative staff, Director and Assistant Director (50–100 percent respectively), and secretary and typist; on-site coordinator; coordinator for each clinical major (50 percent time) and faculty evaluator (14 percent time). Table 13 illustrates personnel costs for one year in each of three outreach programs.

Although the Western Michigan program had the largest number of students and programs, its budget for personnel is the lowest of the three. Inflation is a factor, but also the increase in faculty costs. The HSA VII program reflects the larger number of research-prepared faculty who were outreach teachers. Personnel is the largest budget item in any outreach program, a fact which must be planned for in any outreach budget. It represents almost 68–72 percent of the College of Nursing budgets, but would be less if the community in-kind contributions were included as other budget items.

Program Cost Studies

Two attempts to examine cost of an outreach program were undertaken by the College of Nursing: a one-year cost study during the Western Michigan program and the study of the total cost of the HSA VII program as part of that program's evaluation.

Western Michigan Program

A preliminary study of the cost for the 65 students in the outreach program in Western Michigan for the calendar year 1978–1979 was reported in the American Academy of Nursing publication, *The Impact of Changing Resources on Health Care Policy* (Reilly, 1981). Five cost components were used: compensation for direct instruction, compensation for administration, overhead costs (instructional support), travel, and communication. These components were defined differently than the usual model which includes direct, indirect, and capital costs. Limitations in the accounting system in the university at the time precluded obtaining more definitive data. Table 14 illustrates estimated outreach costs for 1978–1979.

Table 14
Estimated Outreach Costs for 1978–1979

Item	Amount
Compensation for direct instruction	$175,000
Compensation for administration	100,000
Overhead costs	175,000
Travel	18,373
Communication	
Telephone	5,232
Postage	1,852

Compensation for Direct Instruction

There was no difference in direct instructional costs between the on-campus program and outreach program since the teaching assignment used the same work load formula cost per credit hours in each location—$100.00, a sum derived from dividing total salary paid to graduate faculty by credit hours taught, 1,750 in the outreach program.

Compensation for Administration

Administration costs include payment to the administrative staff both on or off campus plus 2 percent of the dean's office staff.

Overhead Costs (Instructional Support Costs)

The formula used at Wayne State University at the time was a ratio 1:1 relative to direct instructional cost and instructional support costs. Since the direct instructional costs was $175,000, instructional support costs were stated as $175,000. The formula recognizes that services and facilities essential for operating a program are already in place, a state which may or may not exist in an outreach program. An example would be a security system for equipment. In the Wayne State University program, it was this category where the in-kind contribution was the greatest for not only were services and facilities provided, they were already in place in the community and thus no such costs were required. The use of the community-based model resulted in a marked decrease in the university's total expenditure of funds of an instructional support cost.

Travel

This category includes travel costs for faculty and staff.

Communication

The money spent on telephone and postage were readily identifiable, but the paper costs, a significant cost item, could not be extrapolated from the university's supply cost data with the accounting system currently in operation at the time.

Although this cost study approach was general in its design, it did present a picture of gross expenditures as they relate to the outreach program. The instructional support costs were minimal because of the model. The extraordinary costs included administration, travel, and communication.

HSA VII Program:
Upper Western, Lower Peninsula, Michigan

Another effort at determining costs of an outreach program involved a retrospective study by the project evaluator to ascertain the cost of the three-year program that was conducted in HSA VII, 256 miles from campus. The cost study included the major categories of direct and indirect costs using the instrument, *Cost of Nursing Education* (National League for Nursing, 1980). The items listed under the two categories were similar to those previously discussed. The capital cost category was not used because no such expenditure was involved.

The study included costs of educational experiences for cognates and electives offered by other institutions of higher learning in the region.

The direct student credit hour cost for nursing course was determined to be $716.00 with the total estimated cost of $812.00. The majority of nursing courses brought to the outreach program were clinical nursing courses which are the most expensive portion of professional graduate programs due to the salary by clinical instructors and other costs associated with clinical practice experiences.

The final report concluded that the per student cost both for credit hour and total costs is directly related to the number of students in the program because the overwhelming proportion associated with the outreach program was assumed to be fixed.

The outreach program in HSA VII was one of the more expensive programs that the College of Nursing offered relative to cost per student for several reasons. Except for the first program, it is the farthest removed from the campus, thus necessitating greater travel costs. Specifically, there was greater use of the more expensive commercial airlines for transporting faculty and staff to the area.

The location of the program in a snow belt area of the state required a modification in the overall planning of the program. Because of the potential for travel difficulties, nursing courses were not brought to the area during the winter term, the only program not offered in a continuous 12-month pattern. Although classes were not in session, the staff and activities of administrators in both the on-campus and off-campus offices needed to be maintained. During the winter term, some students did enroll in cognate or elective courses offered by other institutions in the outreach site.

A third factor was the small enrollment in comparison to other programs. The decision to take the program to the northwestern part of the lower peninsula of Michigan was a deliberate one based on need even though the potential enrollment was limited. The decision was also political, for the College of Nursing was reaching various regions of the state and felt it would be improper to deny this region an opportunity to have some graduate prepared nurses serve its educational and health care settings. Two of the cities in that region were developing medical and health care centers and needed these well-prepared nurse leaders. It must also be noted that concurrent with this program, another 16 students from the College of Nursing were enrolled in an outreach program in the region, Adult Psychiatric and Mental Health Nursing, under separate funds for all clinical courses and the requisite faculty. These students were admitted to some of the non-clinical nursing courses offered in the grant program such as nursing theory, research, and minor courses in administration and teaching. As a result of both programs, a cadre of well-prepared nurses was added to the community. The cost data presented here is based on the students that were in the regular grant supported program.

Lack of comparable data, not only for outreach programs, but for graduate professional programs themselves, limits the ability to interpret any findings. Any retrospective study has its limitations, particularly in data generation. The ability to estimate or determine costs of outreach programs requires a cost accounting system in the institution that permits the appropriate data access and a comparative analysis of findings.

The two approaches to studying costs of these outreach programs are presented for information and not to prescribe an answer to the question, How much does an outreach program cost at the graduate professional level?

CONCLUSION

The costing out of any health professional program is a complex process because of the very nature of such programs which encompass not only the professional and general education components, but also the patient care dimension which contributes to the development of practice skills. The approach to estimating the cost of graduate professional preparation in health fields is even more complex as the research component is incorporated. Without a cost model for these programs, within institutions it is even more difficult to ascertain costs of outreach programs. The major emphasis in this chapter addresses those cost factors relevant to outreach programs.

Questions to be raised by planners of such programs as they estimate costs address the following concerns: mandated services, required contract service, capital costs, equipment, activities that are the responsibility of the institution, activities others can do, particular cost items in outreach programs, and means for augmenting the economic base.

Budgetary items for any outreach program include: personnel (faculty, administrative staff, other), consultation, equipment, supplies, travel, and other. Capital costs may also be an item.

A cost accounting model for estimating the cost of baccalaureate generic nursing programs was proposed as the result of a study by Young (in Kummer, Bednzsh, & Redman, 1987) for the Division of Nursing, Bureau of Health Professions, Health Resources and Services Administration with the American Association of Colleges of Nursing as contractor. The cost components consist of direct, indirect, and capital costs. As a model which addresses the total educational program, it has a potential for use in estimating graduate costs if the research component is provided for in the computation.

One year of the Western Michigan program was examined for costs in relation to five components: compensation for direct instruction, compensation for administration, overhead costs (instructional costs), travel, and communication.

A retrospective study of the HSA VII program conducted by the program evaluator used a model encompassing direct and indirect costs inclusive of all elements of the graduate program. Any study of cost data relative to the College of Nursing programs needs to consider the various sources of financial support, advanced training grant, tuition, in-kind contributions from the community, and service from the university.

9

Outcomes: What Was the Impact of the Outreach Program on the Graduates?

The complexity of processes entailed in providing degree programs in the health professional fields to populations in regions removed from the main campus have been described. The programs represent considerable expenditure of energy, effort, expertise, money, and collaborative ability. But—and this question must be answered—was it worth it?

Any program should have built into its design an evaluation protocol which provides formative data throughout the life of the program and summative data which address its ultimate significance. The character of the data collection and the results obtained are a function of the evaluation questions derived from the stated goals of the endeavor.

Numbers of persons who completed the program or are projected to complete within a reasonable time period following the termination of the program provide some measurement of the degree of success. Numbers reveal little about the quality of the program as it is reflected in the changes in the graduates and the communities where the program existed during its designated time period. The significance of the broader data base in determining outcomes is reinforced in one of the principles in evaluating outreach programs stated by The Council on Postsecondary Accreditation in its Policy Statement on Off-Campus Programs (in Broderius & Carder, 1983):

> Accrediting bodies will place special emphasis on the assessment of outcomes, results, or value-added factors in the evaluation of off-campus

educational activities with respect to institutional program effectiveness and student learning performances.

A comprehensive perspective of impact data is particularly relevant in professional programs where a pattern of behavior as graduates needs to reflect professional persons within both the microsystem of the profession and the macrosystem of the larger society in which they function. Such knowledge is best obtained from follow-up study at several post-program time intervals. The variables examined are derived not only from the patterns of behavior particular to a professional discipline, but also from those behaviors that are characteristic of any professional person within society. A study might include such variables as: perception of self as a professional person, types of employment, continuing education activities, professional organization membership, scholarly productivity, and contribution to the community as citizen and professional. A profile of the graduates based on such variable data and others of particular significance answer the question as to whether the program accomplished its goal of preparing professional practitioners to serve an outreach site.

SOURCES OF COLLEGE OF NURSING OUTCOME DATA

Evaluation Protocol

A rigorous evaluation protocol accompanied the outreach programs in all sites although it was not completely formulated until the end of the first program in the Upper Peninsula. Originally developed by an evaluator from outside Wayne State University, during the last five years the evaluation was the responsibility of a College of Nursing faculty member, Arnold Bellinger, PhD, Associate Professor. In order to maintain a longitudinal study of graduates, the same evaluation forms were continued. The data collected included not only matters addressing the student experience of curriculum elements, but also follow-up studies of graduates and impressions from significant others in the community. Some results from these evaluation reports have been referred to throughout this report. Data discussed at this point are derived from the summary reports that the evaluators completed at the termination of each of the programs. The methods used included questionnaire and interviews with graduates, advisory committee members, and significant other persons on campus and in the outreach site.

Alumnae Study—1986

Much of the outcome data were obtained from the alumnae study of the graduates of the first four programs. The fifth cohort of students was still in the program when this study was initiated. The study was first introduced in the first chapter and subsequent referrals were made to findings throughout the text. Outcome data are the concern of this portion of the report.

An extensive questionnaire seeking quantitative and qualitative data was mailed to 195 graduates (2 graduates are deceased). The objective component related primarily to the five areas of professional behavior: employment patterns, professional organization involvement, advanced study, scholarly activities, and community involvement. The essay component elicited students' perception of the impact of the program on their self-image, goals, and the communities' approach to education and practice of nursing. Any changes noted by the community relative to the image of nursing were also to be noted. The responses to the questionnaire were 154/195 representing 79 percent of the graduates. As with any questionnaire response, on any one question there may be a variation in the number of responses. This fact is particularly noted in the essay questions when some persons do not respond to some or any of the questions. A qualitative result in such questions does not have the same meaning as it does in an objective format; open-ended questions tend to elicit those responses that have a particular meaning to an individual at the time. The exclusion of some response items does not necessarily mean that they were not merited. The numbers of respondents are noted when varying from the expected number.

Other Data

Observable changes in the communities are also included in this report. The communities represent those where the majority of students that were in the program reside.

PROFILE OF GRADUATES

Continued Residence in the Region

One concern often raised in proposing outreach programs is the potential that once the individuals are prepared, they will move from the region. As a result, the goal to upgrade practice in the region through the expertise of well-prepared professionals is illusive. Do outreach graduates move from the region or do outreach programs prepare indigenous residents who remain and contribute to the community? Table 15 illustrates current residence of graduates in Michigan.

Findings from the College of Nursing study suggest that the persons attending their programs were not generally mobile. This result may be a function of the predominating female population in the study wherein women are often attached to a community through family ties, spousal employment, and similar elements. A total of 78 percent of the respondents still reside in Michigan. Four of the respondents moved from one part of the state to another. The

Table 15
Current Residence in Michigan

Program	Respondents	%
Upper Peninsula	12	44
Western Michigan	44	86
HSA VI	35	78
HSA VII	29	94
Total	120	78

greatest mobility is noted for the first group in the Upper Peninsula. This may be related to the time factor, nine years since graduation, but more likely it is related to the changing economic conditions in that region of the state. Many of the spouses of the graduates were employed in either the mining industry or the United States Air Force. With the closing of the mines during the recession period and the inherent mobility of Air Force personnel, some of these graduates left the area because of spousal employment requirements.

Influence of Program on Decision to Earn a MSN

The intent of an outreach program is to reach a population which did not have access to a campus program. Validation of this intent is an important outcome in terms of future planning and justification of the expenditures of money and effort entailed. Table 16 illustrates the influence of a program on graduates' decision to earn a MSN.

The College of Nursing program targeted a group of individuals who would not have earned a Master of Science in Nursing if the programs had not been brought to their regions. Only four respondents planned to earn the degree anyway. The program reached 72 students (47%) who would be unable to earn the degree; many stating family or financial barriers. Those who felt

Table 16
Influence of Program on Graduates'
Decision to Earn a MSN

	Responses No.	%
Anyway	4	3
Unable otherwise	72	47
Eventually later	53	36
Would not have thought of a degree	3	2
Would earn degree outside nursing	45*	29

*Include 23 from unable or eventually.

that they would eventually earn an advanced degree were indefinite about time for such action and a notable 23 out of the 53 who so responded antici- pated that they would earn a degree in a field outside their own discipline. This decision was based on the availability of other types of programs offered in the region. It was not a matter of other choices.

Perceptions of Self

An educational program is directed toward assisting the student in bring- ing about those changes which facilitate the sense of confidence in one's self and the ability to meet the demands of the workplace and the social structure of the environment. This is especially true for graduate professional programs where socialization into a leadership responsibility within the profession is a critical element. With outreach programs at the graduate level, the graduates will constitute the majority of the best-prepared members of the discipline in the region. How one sees oneself is an important element in the person's ability to fulfill the leadership expectations of the community. The College of Nursing sought information from graduates through open-ended questions on two as- pects of self-perception changes: self-image and professional image.

Self-Image. Table 17 illustrates perceived changes in self-image.

In general, a marked increase in self-image was noted in 111 of the responses. Eight responses noted that the program was either "hard on self- image" or resulted in no change. Sample comments are:

See myself as a person with something to contribute.

Program and great faculty influenced my whole life.

Feel good about myself, capabilities, and specialized skills.

Helped me to gain confidence in my abilities to grow and change.

Encouraged me to take risks.

Table 17
Perceived Self-Image Changes ($n = 119$)

Change	No.
Significantly raised	36
Like myself better	22
Confidence—greater independence	15
Now force for change	12
Proud to attain MSN	9
No change	4
WSU program hard on self-image	4

Table 18
Perceived Changes in
Self-Image as a Nurse ($n = 119$)

Change	No.
More confidence with new nursing knowledge	28
See self with more career options, more mobility	19
Increased creditability as a nurse	16
Enhanced sense of professional dedication	9
More proud to be a nurse	9
More qualified to do what I was doing	5

Professional Image.   Table 18 illustrates perceived changes in professional self-image.

New knowledge and competence have greatly enhanced 86 of the responding graduates' perception of themselves as professional nurses. Sample comments are:

Led me to feel good about being a nurse.

Different image of self—less a follower, more a leader.

Seen as creditable professional nurse with wealth of knowledge and skills.

Feel very confident in my clinical role.

Now I am qualified for what I was doing.

Goals

What happens to student goals when they enter a graduate program? Individuals in outreach sites often far removed from the stimulation of the major learning centers in their field may have very limited goals which are more or less defined by the community where they practice. New horizons and career potentials are often the result of the nature of the studies themselves and the experiences which the campus faculty share with the students and the kind of professional model they represent. This fact was particularly noted by one graduate who has since earned a PhD in Nursing. "I had never thought of graduate school or a university career until my 'eyes were opened' and able to see an entirely new, diverse world through participation in the MSN courses and exposure to new and different world views. If the outreach program had not come to the *region*, I believe I would still be living there and working as a staff nurse in the ICU."

Goal change does not require moving from the community for greater opportunities, but rather it can provide a challenge to the graduates to modify practice and to be pioneers in introducing new roles and practices in the community. The latter can often be realized because graduates are of that region and thus are known and accepted. In addition, because their clinical practice has been in the community, their new ideas have already been introduced. Table 19 illustrates perceived goal changes.

The graduates' responses denote that the program impacted on goals in two main ways: expanded their goals or facilitated goal achievement.

Sample comments are:

Goals are higher and expectations greater.

Haven't changed significantly—ability to attain goals has changed immensely.

Opened doors for me that I never would have dreamed would open.

Developed goals and desires to pursue a career rather than a job.

Without MSN would likely leave nursing and pursue social work. Love what I am doing.

Stimulated me to go for higher degree.

Employment

Graduate programs, especially in outreach sites, have as a mission the preparation of leaders to assist the community move its practices forward. In a profession such as nursing, preparation at the master's level is appropriate for leadership roles. Although doctoral preparation in nursing is the highest level, the percentage of nurses having earned this academic achievement at this time is less than 1 percent. Therefore, graduate study at the master's level is the present mode for preparing nursing leaders particularly in regions removed from the major centers of nursing education and practice.

Leadership positions in professional fields are generally classed as: administrator (service or education), teacher, and clinical specialist. In the smaller communities, these positions are often filled by individual nurses with undergraduate preparation in nursing in another field, for they are the only resource available. An outreach professional program not only prepares

Table 19
Perceived Goal Changes ($n = 120$)

Change	No.
Expand goal expectations	44
No change-facilitated achievement	17
Changed view of nursing	13
Moved from job to career	10
Influenced chosen career for a lifetime	5
Encouraged to seek and gain PhD	4

individuals for those leadership roles, but must also prepare those persons already holding such positions so that they can be more effective in fulfilling the responsibilities entailed in the position. Figure 6 depicts positions held by graduates before and after the MSN program.

Data indicate that 86 percent of graduates (132/154) are in leadership positions. Of note are the 111 who were in such positions prior to the program without adequate preparation. An additional 21 prepared graduates joined the leadership group. There is a significant increase in the number of nurses who moved into leadership positions. The shift in positions following the program were from staff nurse to leadership roles. The unemployed graduates were students in a doctorate program, between positions, or meeting family demands with several having new born infants. Table 20 illustrates positions held by outreach graduates and currently.

The shift was toward increase in administrator, inservice educators, and clinical specialists. The decrease in number of faculty is somewhat misleading, for some of the faculty at entry are now in administrative positions as directors of nursing schools. Of the 148 who responded to the question relative to the place of employment, 50 percent (74) stated they were working in schools of nursing while another 35 percent (51) were working in hospitals.

Figure 6
Positions Held by Graduates before
and after the MSN Program

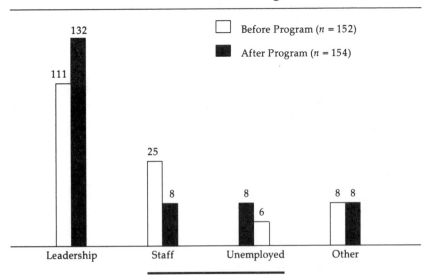

Table 20
Positions Held by Outreach Graduates and Currently

Position	Employment at Entry		Currently	
	No.	%	No.	%
Faculty	66	44	57	37
Administrator	24	16	33	21
Inservice educator	15	10	25	16
Clinical specialist	6	4	17	11
Staff	25	16	8	5
Unemployed	8	5	6	4
Other	8	5	8	5
Total	152		154	

Graduates cited 14 reasons why they changed positions, but the majority of responses were in several categories. The ranking of these reasons is noted in Table 21.

Sample comments from graduates relative to the impact of the outreach program on their employment patterns are:

Showed me I could do whatever I wanted and has encouraged me to go on and do other things.

Able to apply for and get position as specialist.

Allowed me to have the best of both worlds—teaching/practice.

Could not hold present position without degree.

Able to accomplish goal of collaborative practice within five months, not five years.

Table 21
Ranking of Reasons for Change in
Position after MSN Program

Reason	UP	WM	HSA VI	HSA VII
Advancement	1	1	1	1
Greater opportunity	4 (a)	2	2	4(b)
Need for new experience	3	3	3	3
(a) UP	—2nd ranked reason = spouse relocation			
(b) HSAV II	—2nd ranked reason = more compatible with preparation			

The influence of the outreach program on the present position was noted by 66 percent of the respondents with only 7 percent feeling that there was no impact.

In response to the question of whether the current position is compatible with the professional goal, 70/147 were satisfied. Of the 77 respondents whose present positions were incongruent with their goals, 20 were seeking positions as faculty, administrators, or researchers and 16 did not provide a goal. An interesting trend was noted in the response of 34 persons who were looking for a career which combined at least two roles. The predominating combination was teaching and practice (22 respondents), an increasingly recommended career pattern for nursing so that faculty maintain their practice skills and contribute their knowledge and expertise to the delivery of nursing services. Teaching and research roles in a combined position were the choice of five other persons with one respondent wanting a position that combined the roles of teaching, practice, and research. This trend of looking for positions which combine several roles is relatively recent in nursing. When alumnae were studied in 1981, there was no mention of dual positions.

When respondents were asked to indicate deterrents to their reaching employment goals, 12 reasons were cited. The four reasons receiving the highest response were: limited opportunity in the area (71), personal family (31), more advanced study needed (21), and lack of mobility (20).

One other significant dimension of the employment factor is the financial remuneration which graduates can expect after completing a program of studies. While there are many elements inclusive to a payment formula, it is important for outreach planners to consider the relationship between salary and geographical location. The income increase of the outreach graduates of the College of Nursing Master of Science in Nursing program was noted by 102/151 respondents while another 49 stated that they had received no increase in income. The two major reasons cited by the latter group were: (1) set pay scale and (2) no recognition of their new preparation. Table 22 illustrates range of increase in income since graduation.

Most graduates reported an increase in their yearly income of between $1,000 and $5,000 dollars. There is also significant correlation between length of time since graduation and increase in income (Spearman .24, $p \leq .007$).

Table 22
Range of Increase in
Income since Graduation

Income Increase	Respondents	%
0–999	13	13
1–4,999	49	48
5–9,999	21	21
10,000+	19	23
	$n = 102$	

Among the most recent graduates (HSA VII), 30 percent reported an increase of less than $1,000 while only 5 percent of the graduates in the first program (UP) had such an increase. The opposite trend for income increase is noted for over $10,000. Income increase appears to be minimal at first with potential for greater amounts in the long term.

Membership in Professional Organizations

Identification with one or more professional organizations is an expected behavior of a professional. Membership can represent varied forms and degrees of participation, but it does signify a commitment to the profession and to its efforts both to serve its members and serve society which provides it the license to practice. The official professional organization in nursing is the American Nurses' Association, but within the profession there are other types of organizations such as those concerned with the various clinical practice specialities. Nurses also belong to other organizations which are composed of various professionals focusing on a particular health concern.

Membership in the American Nurses' Association has not been remarkably high among nurses. A notation in the Institute of Medicine study, *Nursing and Nursing Education* (1983, p. 41), states that in 1982 only 10 percent of the nurses who hold licenses to practice were members of their professional organization. Various factors may account for this finding. Most nurses are married females who historically have placed their professional activities as secondary to the professional needs of their spouses. Many nurses also are not prepared at the professional educational level found in other disciplines, and thus the values associated with professional membership may have not been as well articulated or perceived. Other factors are also operating in this situation, but present trends suggest that professional membership will increase as the educational level of nurses increase and women in the work place of nursing become more career and less job oriented.

The professional membership profile of the graduates of the Master of Science in Nursing Outreach Program is illustrated in Table 23.

This group of graduates meets the criterion of professional membership to a remarkable degree, 90 percent holding membership in some professional

Table 23
Professional Organization Membership
of Graduates before and after
Completion of MSN Program

Membership	Respondents before	after	%
Yes	122	139	90
No	32	15	10
	154	154	

organization with distribution generally consistent among graduates of all groups. This figure represents an increase of 17 respondents (11 percent) since completing the program. No previous membership in any organization was noted by 21 percent (32) respondents. McNemar statistic for correlated proportions was significant—p ≤ .0001. regarding those who had membership before and those who had membership after. Table 24 illustrates major professional organizations in which graduates hold membership.

Membership in the American Nurses' Association is held by 73 percent (113/154). At the time of entry into the program, 50 percent (77) of the graduates were members. During or after the program, 16 withdrew membership but 51 new graduates became members. McNemar test for correlated proportions was highly significant—p ≤ .0001. These figures are remarkably high if one considers as a basis the estimated 10 percent of all registered nurses who belong to this professional organization.

The second highest percentage, 51 (79/154), of membership is in Sigma Theta Tau, International Nursing Honorary Society. The 22 percent membership (34/154) in clinical speciality organization reflects a trend which will continue in the future as nurses seek colleagueship with other nurses in the same area of clinical practice.

Most graduates, 53 percent (81/154), belong to 1–2 organizations with another 34 percent (54/154) belonging to 3–5 organizations. Positions of responsibility in these organizations are noted by 49 percent (73/149), a generally consistent distribution among all 4 groups.

Several factors must be noted here. These graduates were already involved in professional organizations before the outreach program came to their region. This finding may reflect a social phenomenon in outreach sites where professionals tend to get together in organizational meetings for support, education, and colleagueship since they are often isolated from other avenues of professional activities which are found in the larger metropolitan areas. The increased involvement of these graduates as a result of the outreach program is noted in some of the graduates' comments:

Makes me want to fight harder for nursing.

Increased my involvement in my profession tremendously.

Table 24
Major Professional Organizations in which Graduates Hold Memberships

Type	Respondents	%
American Nurses' Association	113	73
National League for Nursing	26	18
Sigma Theta Tau	80	51
Practice speciality	34	22
Interdisciplinary	22	14

Extended goals to becoming politically active in shaping future of professional nursing.

Now have strong values relative to professional organizations, professional education, etc.

See potential to make a significant impact on nursing locally.

Advanced Study

A professional behavior is the pattern for continuing education both to meet academic qualifications for specific responsibilities in the field and to maintain a level of professional competency within an everchanging practice. Further educational activities may include formal studies leading to an advanced degree, studies leading to certification in a speciality area of practice, or participation in conferences and programs which address issues and practices in the field.

Doctoral Study

Doctoral study in nursing is a relatively new phenomenon. The first doctorate program in nursing was established in 1961 at the University of Pittsburgh. Two doctoral degrees are now awarded: Doctor of Philosophy and Doctor of Nursing Science. Both are research degrees which include study in nursing and related fields.

Prior to the establishment of doctoral programs in nursing, nurses earned doctorate degrees in education, public health, and science disciplines relevant to nursing's body of knowledge, that is, physiology, biology, microbiology, anthropology, sociology, and psychology. The trend now is for nurses to enter doctoral studies in their own discipline.

Doctoral study is now a goal in the plan of an increasing number of nurses as they enter graduate study. A sample of some of the comments made by the respondents in the College of Nursing Master of Science in Nursing Outreach Program follows:

Prepared me for doctoral study.

Committed to a professional career—plan a doctorate.

Encouraged me to reach further, am now a PhD student.

At the time the data for the alumnae study were collected, six of the respondents had completed their doctoral study and another 19 were enrolled in doctoral programs. One of the graduates not included in this study died shortly after completing her PhD degree in nursing. As of this writing, one of the "in-progress" graduates completed her PhD degree in nursing.

Table 25
Reasons Why Graduates Choose to
Earn a Doctorate Degree

Reasons	No.	% of Respondents
Professional stimulation	59	44
New opportunities	51	38
Advancement in position	18	13
Economic advancement	3	2
Prepare for research	2	2
Job security	2	2

The distribution of doctoral degrees among the 25 respondents are PhD in Nursing (10), Doctor of Nursing Science (1), Doctorate in another field (9), Doctor of Education (5).

Another 47 percent (60/128) respondents plan to enroll in doctoral study, with 55 percent currently planning to earn a doctorate degree in nursing. Nine respondents are not sure as to what field they will pursue. Reasons cited for pursuing a doctorate degree were cited by 135 respondents (see Table 25).

The predominant reason for continuing study at the doctoral level was for professional stimulation while the opportunity for new experiences is a close second.

Certification

Currently 24 percent (37/154) of the respondents are certified in ten areas of nursing with four predominating areas: critical care nursing (9), psychiatric and mental health nursing (8), nursing administration (7), maternity nursing (6).

Another 18 respondents have earned post-master certificate representing eight different areas. The most frequent areas were: gerentologic nursing (7), critical care nursing (3), and administration (3).

Attendance at Conferences

Provisions for continuing education are very much a part of the professional pattern of the respondents to the alumnae study. A total of 88 percent (123/140) have attended conferences or workshops since graduation with 53 percent (74/154) attending five or more sessions.

Graduates are pursuing their education within three major modes: programs leading to a degree, certification in a special area, or attendance at programs and other types of continuing education activities. The direction of the study and the timing of the activity are functions of the time since graduation. Most of the doctoral students are drawn from the first two groups with seven of the third group so involved and certification is primarily achieved by graduates of the first three programs, but four of the last group have met the criteria.

Scholarly Productivity

Graduates of professional programs at the graduate level have a responsibility not only to provide leadership in the dissemination of professional knowledge so as to influence the practice, but also to become generators of the knowledge attributed to a field. Research expertise in this country is generally acknowledged to be within the province of those members of a profession with an earned doctorate degree where much of the development of research skills is emphasized. However, master's programs do incorporate a research component and some of the graduates do engage in research activities. Comments from some of the students suggest the impact of the research activity in the master's program:

Sparked my interest in research.

Will have research published.

Aspirations to write nursing article.

Provided credentials for authorship of a book.

In the graduate group under study, 44 out of 153 respondents have been or are currently engaged in research activities. The majority are drawn from the first three programs, but it is interesting to note that five of the most recent graduates are already involved. Most of the studies are being funded by the employing institution, 54 percent, a significant trend since funding for nursing research by a health agency is a recent activity. Other sources of funding include health organizations in the community, other community groups, and the Division of Nursing, Bureau of Health Resources and Health Administration for two graduates. Seven respondents were conducting their study without any outside funding.

Publication is a domain of scholarly activity expected of professionals. Two graduates have published books in their field, and two others have published in refereed professional journals while another 12 graduates have been published in nonrefereed journals. Other types of publications include: abstracts, monographs, proceedings, or manuals. A total of 29 respondents have been published.

Presentations at professional meetings is another behavior characteristic of professionals in a field. Fifty percent (73/144) of the respondents have presented before professional groups. Within the 50 percent one or two presentations were given by 65 percent (48); 13 percent (10) gave three to four presentations; and 10 percent (7) gave five to six presentations. Of particular note are the five graduates who have delivered over 15 presentations.

Twenty-seven graduates have been awarded honors: ten from groups in their community, nine from the university or health agency where they are employed, two from their district nurses association, and one from the Michigan Nurses Association.

Community Involvement

Professional activities of individuals extend beyond those of the immediate work place to the enhancement of the health and welfare of their community. In an outreach program, students maintain usual residences and designated community roles and also use the resources of the community for their field practice. Upon graduation, therefore, the students continue to be accepted in their communities. The customary opportunities to participate in varied activities and assist with changes directed toward the community's health are enhanced by the educational preparation.

An examination of the quality of a program includes data relative to the community contributions of its graduates. Such information was sought from the College of Nursing outreach graduates: 78 percent (120/154) of the graduates are actively involved with groups concerned about community health matters. Involvement in community activities is positively related to time since graduation—Spearman $r = .16$, $p \leq .02$. Table 26 illustrates types of community activities in which graduates are involved.

Teaching is the major community activity with board and committee membership second. As one student stated, "The program enabled me to enter the community at the policy, decision-making level." The other categories included such activities as guardian in a juvenile court, lobbyist, consultant, and developer of programs and special clinics.

Students commented on the influence of the outreach program on their present professional role in the community:

Broadened my perspective of health care and how I might impact.

Much more visible in the community.

Table 26
Types of Community Activities in
which Graduates Are Involved

Type of Activity	Responses
Teaching health to groups	94
Board membership	54
Teaching special groups	48
Leading group session	46
Contributing to media	31
Committee membership	5
Other	13

Became more aware of health concerns—thought they were someone else's concern.

Learned community service is essential part of professional life.

More active role in health concerns.

COMPARISON OF PROFESSIONAL
PROFILE OF TWO GROUPS ADMITTED

It was noted (see chapter 1) that there were two groups of students admitted to the College of Nursing outreach program: one represented students who met the criterion of graduation from a National League for Nursing accredited baccalaureate program and one represented students whose baccalaureate program was either from a non-accredited baccalaureate nursing program or a non-nursing program. The decision to accept students who do not meet the baccalaureate program criterion is debated in numerous professional arenas. However, it is a recognized fact that in many outreach sites leadership positions are filled by individuals without the requisite preparation. To deny them access to an advanced program would deter a group of nurses already involved in their field from preparing themselves appropriately for present and future role demands. The action could also create political issues which might interfere with the successful outcome of the outreach endeavor. Although accepting such individuals may be perceived by some as lowering the standards of nursing, one might also see these admissions as an opportunity to raise the standard of nursing by preparing these individuals and bringing them into the mainstream of nursing.

Because the College of Nursing made provisions for these persons who did not meet this entry criterion to address some of their deficiencies and validate their nursing knowledge as appropriate to enter graduate study, the data analysis included an examination of each of these two groups on professional criteria using a chi square test of significance. On all professional items there was no significant difference between the groups. In presenting the data the two groups are identified as: *Group A*, those graduates who met the criterion of graduation from accredited nursing baccalaureate programs, and *Group B*, those graduates who did not meet the criterion.

The number of graduates in each group is;

Group A	101	66%
Group B	53	34%
Total	154	

Slightly more of Group B graduates still reside in Michigan, 83 percent (44/53), than do Group A graduates, 76 percent (76/101). Likewise, the presence of the program in the outreach site influenced the Group B students to obtain a master's degree in nursing to a greater extent. No graduate in Group B felt that he or she would obtain the degree anyway while four in Group A indicated that this action was likely. In Group B, 57 percent (30/53) stated that without the program they would not be able to earn the master's degree in nursing. This feeling was expressed by 42 percent (42/101) of Group A graduates.

Employment data support the assumption at the beginning of the program that many leadership positions in nursing in the community would be filled by persons who did not meet the entry criterion of graduation from an accredited baccalaureate program. In the leadership category, at time of entry, 86 percent (44/51) Group B graduates were so employed. Of particular note is the 53 percent (27/51) who were faculty in schools of nursing. Most of these students continued on in two major functional areas of leadership, teaching and administration, when they graduated.

Congruency exists in the responses of both groups relative to academic pursuits after graduation: 4 percent of each group completed a doctorate degree and another 12 percent are in doctoral programs.

Participation in professional organizations is intense for both groups with 87 percent (88/101) of Group A and 96 percent (51/53) of Group B holding membership in a nursing organization. Group B graduates have slightly higher membership in the American Nurses' Association, 81 percent (43/53) vs. 70 percent (70/101), and the National League of Nursing, 23 percent (23/53) vs. 14 percent (14/101). This difference might be anticipated since many were already in leadership positions prior to entry into the program and could have established a professional network.

There are no significant differences in the profile of the graduates, regardless of the group to which they belong. Several factors may account for this finding. The Group B students were more self-selected since they had to meet prerequisites before being admitted. The prerequisite demands eliminated those applicants who could not meet the academic criteria or who lacked the motivation to address their deficits. Also, as was noted earlier, many of Group B graduates were already professionally involved in nursing in their communities and had previously been motivated to seek whatever education was available to them in their community. Once the students were admitted, the program itself became an equalizer.

Because of the decision to accommodate nurses who did not meet the entry criteria relative to type of baccalaureate preparation, periodic studies were conducted during the first three programs to determine if there was a difference in the academic performance between the two groups. The quality point average was used as the criterion with 3.0 required for graduation. Data were based on academic performance at the time of graduation, thus the total numbers do not reflect all the graduates from any one program since some students delayed their completion date. The findings showed remarkable consistency in the mean average: Group A = 3.62 and Group B = 3.60. The group delineation for quality point average was not continued in the fourth program.

The profile of the graduates who did not possess all requisites for admission demonstrate highly professionally socialized graduates who now continue in the community with the preparation essential for fulfillment of inherent leadership responsibilities.

PROFILE OF PROFESSIONAL NURSES

Data reported provide a qualitative dimension to the evaluation of the outreach program. They provide evidence that the program addressed not only the need for increased numbers of nurses with a master's degree in their discipline, but also the need for these individuals to be professionally socialized in order to provide the leadership essential for the community's ability to serve the health care needs of its constituents.

It is this ability to prepare such a professionally oriented person that is often challenged when professional programs are offered in their total away from the main campus. The profile of the 154 graduates in this study demonstrate that the outreach program can meet the goal of professional socialization.

The graduates note with satisfaction a major increase in professional and personal self-image as well as evolving goals. Objectively, shifts to more leadership positions, increase in income, number of memberships in professional organizations, and involvement in community health concerns were noted. Graduates exhibited a high level of scholarly activity which included doctoral study, research, publication, and presentations at professional meetings.

This change is reflected in activities with leadership positions as faculty, administrators, and clinical specialists currently held by 86 percent. About half of the graduates are in positions congruent with their goals while some students want either to combine roles, particularly teaching and practice, or become established in one of the leadership roles such as teacher, clinical specialist, or administrator.

Professional orientation is reflected in their extensive involvement in professional organizations. Advancement in scholarly pursuits is evident in the movement toward doctoral study, particularly the PhD in nursing, which is seen as fulfilling the need for professional stimulation. It is further exemplified by the large numbers presenting papers at professional meetings and the beginning evidence of authorship and research.

Increased awareness of community health concerns and the role nurses can play has led to involvement by over 78 percent of the graduates in teaching, leading groups, and membership on boards and committees of local agencies.

The description of the data analysis just presented portrays an involved, confident, goal-directed nursing leader contributing both to the profession and to the community.

Professional socialization in an outreach program does not just happen, however. Rather it is the result of deliberately planning the program with that goal in mind. Examination of the process from student and faculty comments provides clues. In addition to the very nature of the graduate program itself, faculty were a major contributor to this process. Except in rare instances, all nursing courses were taught by senior College of Nursing faculty, the same faculty who taught courses on campus. As role models, such faculty were already involved as professionals at the local, state, national, and international levels of action and were demonstrated scholars through their research and publications.

A concentrated period of faculty–student interaction was provided through the pattern of the program—every third weekend for a course involving Friday evenings and Saturdays. Opportunities to share in a common experience of travel and to have meals together resulted in a spirit of camaraderie. Faculty then became significant socializing agents for professional development.

An additional factor was the close network established among students who were all sharing the same experience. They became a source of support for one another as the demands for change in behavior and outlook became evident.

The study did not address comparative professional behavior between on-campus and off-campus students. After the first two programs were completed, the evaluator did look at the two groups on some of the same variables. He reported that outreach students showed higher scores on the variables. The resources for continuing such an evaluation study were not available and thus the major concern became whether or not professional socialization did occur as evidenced by certain manifestations accepted in the literature as significant in assessing professional behavior.

CONCLUSION

A qualitative assessment of an outreach endeavor extends far beyond the report of numbers of students who earned a degree. Quality involves other factors that address the performance of graduates in accord with stated objectives of the program, the delivery of a program not only consistent with the policies and procedures of the student population, and the impact of such an endeavor on the graduates, the community involved, and the institutional sponsor.

The Master of Science in Nursing program of the College of Nursing, Wayne State University, maintained a formative and summative evaluation protocol which addressed varied qualitative elements. Of great significance was program impact on the professional socialization of the graduates as leaders so as to provide direction to nursing in teaching, practice, and administration. Professional socialization is a major objective of the graduate program of the college and its attainment is critical if its graduates are to influence nursing in their respective communities. In evaluating the graduates, professional behavior variables were used, including: perception of self as a person and nurse, present and future career goals, types of employment, continuing education activities, professional organization memberships, scholarly productivity, and contributions to the health and welfare of the community as citizen and as professional.

Further data analysis indicated a consistency in the professional profile of graduates who met entry criterion of graduation from a baccalaureate program in nursing which was accredited by the National League for Nursing and those whose baccalaureate degree was earned in another type of program. Many educators question the ability of nurses to proceed to a graduate level nursing program if the baccalaureate preparation was not in nursing. Findings in this study suggest that the students not meeting the requisite criterion are self-selected and have a strong motivation factor in operation. To be admitted, the students were required to validate their nursing knowledge and address deficits from the previous program. Once in the program, the program itself became an equalizer offering the same opportunities to all students.

On all criteria, the outreach graduate profile was outstanding and involvement of the graduates as change agents is remarkable and evident in all dimensions of nursing. Professional socialization can occur even though the total graduate program is offered away from the main campus, but there must be a deliberate, conscious effort by all involved to assure that students will indeed reflect professional behavior on the completion of the program.

10

Outcomes: What Was the Impact of the Outreach Program in the Communities Involved?

A quality assessment of an outreach program is concerned not only with the graduates of the program, but also with the communities themselves where the program was located or where the graduates practice. A program situated in an area for a designated period of time becomes part of that community and thus has the opportunity to assist in the development of the community. Likewise, the community should feel the influence of a group of well-prepared individuals when their services are made available.

The latter statement is particularly true when professional programs are offered in outreach sites since the paramount reason for bringing such programs is to prepare indigenous persons to serve their community. The Master of Science in Nursing Outreach Program, which the College of Nursing brought to five regions in the state, was perceived as a "mass inoculation" of a community whereby a cadre of nurses would be prepared at a graduate level for leadership. When the college completed the program and withdrew from the community, these nurses would then provide the necessary leadership to bring about the desired changes. Did this mass inoculation result in changes in the community?

In examining a community, longitudinal studies are important, for time is a significant factor in any major change. The evaluators of the outreach program included interview data from individuals in the various communities and the alumnae of the program relative to their perception of the meaning of the program to their community. A wider variety of individuals were interviewed in the first two programs because the outreach endeavor was a new enterprise and validation of the effort was sought. Formative evaluation was also essential as the program moved into different regions. The latter programs sought data from a limited population, primarily the members of the advisory committee, the on-site coordinator, and students. Incorporated in the evaluation protocol were questions that addressed impact of the program on the community.

Further data were obtained in the 1986 alumnae study where graduates responded to an open-ended question relative to their perceptions of the impact of the program on nursing education in their communities, the perception of nursing held by individuals in their communities, and nursing service. Objective data were also obtained through observation of changes.

CHANGES IN COMMUNITIES
AFTER CLOSURE OF MSN PROGRAM

Upper Peninsula Program

A case method of evaluation was used in evaluating the Upper Peninsula program at its closure, December, 1977. Incorporated in that study was an interview schedule for obtaining data from the college presidents and the directors of nursing in the two major institutions: Northern Michigan University and Lake Superior State College. All agreed that the most critical issue in this remote area of the state was the need to prepare faculty so that the quality of the programs in the region could be enhanced and the nursing programs could be accredited by the National League for Nursing. There was also concern that the nursing faculty preparation was far inferior to their colleagues in other departments in the institutions. It was felt that the advancement of nursing in the region could not proceed without the leadership of a well-prepared faculty who could influence the direction that those whom they taught would take in practice.

At the conclusion of the second program, the evaluator returned to the Upper Peninsula (two years after the program closed there) and found universal agreement by faculty, graduates, and community leaders who were interviewed that the program helped to get nurses with advanced degrees into this isolated area and that a high quality of assistance to nurses at all levels was achieved. Both faculty and practitioners noted change in two significant areas: morale and prestige of nurses were enhanced.

Marked changes have occurred in the Upper Peninsula area since the outreach program terminated. The community position that movement in nursing depended first on acquiring a well-prepared faculty was well founded and the improvement in health care services resulted from the attainment of this goal through the Master of Science in Nursing program.

At the onset of the program two institutions provided baccalaureate education for nursing, Northern Michigan University and Lake Superior State College. The latter also had an Associate Degree in Nursing program. Because neither school had prepared faculty, they were unable to obtain either state approval or national accreditation. Now ten years later, both schools are not only state approved, they also have their programs accredited by the National League for Nursing.

In addition, Northern Michigan University received a grant from the Division of Nursing, USDHHS to begin a Master of Science in Nursing program. The first program with a track in nursing administration began in 1985; a clinical track in nursing care of the adult is also beginning. A faculty, that at one time had only six individuals with a master's degree (most not in nursing), now is chaired by a nurse with a PhD in nursing and has several faculty with doctorate degrees and several currently in doctoral programs. The school now has an outreach program located in several sites in the Upper Peninsula to assist nurses who wish to continue their studies to obtain a bachelor's degree in nursing.

Lake Superior State College continues to meet the needs of nurses in the eastern part of the Upper Peninsula and Saulte Ste. Marie, Ontario. The director of the nursing program is in a doctorate program as are several faculty.

Leadership in the region is evident from both institutions. Faculty are involved in health groups in the community, provide continuing education to nurses, actively participate in the local and state nursing organizations, and sponsor periodic research conferences.

Some of the outreach graduates are providing leadership in practice and hold joint appointments in a school of nursing and a health care agency. Following the program, there appeared the first clinical specialists prepared at the graduate level. Other nurses are now consultants to health agencies.

Nursing is indeed alive and well in the Upper Peninsula, the region of the state where the College of Nursing first brought its Master of Science in Nursing Outreach Program. The region is now in the position of generating its own nurses at the graduate level, a goal the Wayne State University College of Nursing cited in its first grant application. Nurses are held in high esteem not only in their community, but throughout the state and the delivery of nursing care has been greatly enhanced through the efforts of the early graduates and the nurses whom they teach.

Western Michigan Program

The first study of the impact of the Master of Science in Nursing Outreach Program on the community in Western Michigan was conducted by the evaluator at the conclusion of the program in December, 1979. At that time, interviews with nursing leaders and selected graduates revealed their strong belief that the outreach program was essential for the advancement of nursing and nursing education. At that early stage, they already saw advantages to the program: faculty were being promoted once they were prepared, colleagues of the graduates were seeing "new life" in their profession, more interest was expressed relative to the nursing literature, and sophistication at a professional level was evident to some. All concurred that such a program was essential to prepare nurses in the community because recruitment in that area from outside the region had limited possibilities.

When the program evaluator sought data from the graduates one year after they completed their program, it was found that many of the responders were employed in academic positions, and that they had a high involvement in the professional nurses organizations and in research activity.

There have been marked changes in the region since the program terminated, December, 1979. When the program came to the site, education for nurses occurred primarily in hospital schools of nursing. There were several community colleges and two baccalaureate programs, Grand Valley State College and Nazareth College. During the period that the program was in the region, the Grand Valley State College's baccalaureate program received accreditation from the National League for Nursing.

Seven years later, all but one of the six hospital-based schools of nursing have been closed. A new baccalaureate program in nursing was established under the egis of two colleges, Hope-Calvin, and, as a result, the Butterworth hospital school of nursing closed. The Hackley hospital school of nursing in Muskegon closed and the associate degree program in Muskegon Community College opened. The St. Mary's hospital school of nursing closed and is now a setting for the outreach baccalaureate program from Mercy College in Detroit. Ferris State College in Big Rapids was offering a practical nursing program and an associate nursing program, all unaccredited. It has since discontinued its practical nursing program and now has a two-level program which provides for associate and baccalaureate students. The college has also reached out into the community by offering an outreach baccalaureate nursing program to nurses who do not have such a degree and has also developed a health center which provides for ambulatory nursing care to individuals in the community and serves as a practice site for its students and faculty.

There have also been changes in the practice of nursing in the region. One of the most noted changes was the introduction of the clinical nurse specialists, especially in the hospitals. One administrator made the following comment to the director, "You at Wayne State University have shown us what we didn't know we could have. We have hired some clinical specialists who graduated from the outreach program and now we want more. Therefore, we need to generate our own specialists." These graduates sold themselves and their expertise. One of the graduates convinced a community agency whose focus was on needs of the elderly to hire her, for the staff was primarily composed of social workers and psychologists. She not only demonstrated the role of the nurse, but also increased the complement of nurses on the staff. Now hospitals and other health agencies are employing clinical nurse specialists. Some graduates are now in executive leadership positions in hospitals and public health agencies while others are engaged as entrepreneurs offering their own particular nursing services.

A spin off of this program was the decision to bring the last outreach program of the College of Nursing to southwestern Michigan, 60 miles from where the western program was held. In the western program there was a group of students from the Kalamazoo area who had provided remarkable leadership in the Southwestern Michigan community of nurses. The climate had so changed that a master's degree in nursing had become the accepted credential for leadership positions in teaching, administration, and practice. A high research orientation was evident among nursing groups in the community with many nurses doing their own studies and an annual research conference offered by a consortium of nurses from the local hospitals and nursing schools. There was no master's program in the region, so the College of Nursing responded to the request of this highly motivated group of nurses.

As was true for the first program, the Western Michigan program has resulted in many changes in the community, again influencing the morale of the nurses with their new found self-confidence and the prestige of the nurses as they demonstrate their expertise in all domains of nursing. Like the first program, alterations in educational practice in the community was the primary change focus—other changes came about as a result of this focus. An additional effect has been the recognition of the professional climate for nursing in these communities which facilitates their efforts to recruit nurses from outside their regions.

HSA VI Program (Mideastern Michigan)

Changes are less remarkable here in comparison to the previous two programs. This program (HSA VI) was completed in December, 1981. At that time, interviews were held by the program evaluator with the director of the health center where the program was located and the community advisory committee. The respondents saw the program as having a significant impact in meeting the needs of the community, especially for master's-prepared nurse faculty. Although the need for nursing administrators prepared at the graduate level was evident, this fact was not acknowledged by the hospital nursing administrators who were interviewed. Since many did not have such preparation, this absence may well be in response to their own job security concerns. The public health nursing administrator felt there was a need for administrators in that area of nursing to be prepared at the graduate level.

In the summer of 1983, the evaluator sought follow-up data from the graduates through an alumnae questionnaire. It was noted that many of the respondents were employed in administration positions rather than in academic ones, a notable shift from the findings of the previous two programs. This was also an interesting finding in light of the advisory committee members perception that the need was greatest for faculty and less for administrators. One other difference was noted in the response of these graduates from

that of previous ones; earlier graduates saw the outreach program as contributing toward such actions as their promotion or merit raises, these later
alumnae saw the program as a means of maintaining their present position.

Since the program was terminated, the Saginaw Valley School of Nursing received accreditation for its baccalaureate nursing program from the
National League for Nursing and is seeking permission to develop a master's
degree program in nursing. The outreach program provided faculty for the
school while other graduates became clinical nursing specialists. Several
graduates became entrepreneurs and incorporated their business. They now
serve as consultants to health care agencies and carry out such activities as
health screening for various communities and schools.

HSA VII Program
(Upper Northwestern Lower Peninsula)

In the fourth program which was completed in February, 1985, some
trends for change are evident. The evaluator of the program held interviews
with nursing leaders, selected students, and the advisory committee members
to obtain their perception of the potential impact of the outreach program in
their community. When the program entered the region, there was only one
faculty member in the local community college nursing department with a
master's degree in nursing. (She was a graduate of the first outreach program.)
Many faculty attended the outreach program and the community college was
then in a position to require that all nursing faculty must be prepared at the
master's level. The community college in Petoskey, north of Traverse City, also
received the benefit of prepared faculty as some of the graduates sought employment in that institution.

In the local hospitals, the directors stated that in the future a master's-
prepared nurse would be employed in the leadership positions. One of the
outreach graduates was appointed to a newly created hospital position as
oncology nurse specialist; more clinical nursing specialist roles are now
evolving in the region and the interviews elicited information that such roles
would increase particularly in the rural ambulatory service agencies. One
graduate introduced the clinical nursing specialist role in a cooperative practice with a physician. The physician and nurse now have clinics in two different rural areas and both have hospital privileges in a neighboring city. Their
clientele is primarily women with emphasis on those who are pregnant.

Movement is evident in this community even though the time span since
the program completion is only two years.

ALUMNAE PERCEPTIONS OF
CHANGES IN THEIR COMMUNITIES

In the alumnae study of 1986, the 120 respondents who were still residing in
the communities where they attended the outreach program were requested

to answer an open-ended question on the questionnaire. This question focused on perceived changes in their community in the realms of education, nursing service, and the community's image of nursing. A content analysis resulted in the identification of the major themes which occurred in the responses.

Nursing Education

As might be expected, the change most frequently acknowledged was the improvement in the quality of faculty in the schools of nursing. This change resulted in the improved quality of education of students, the increase in the scope of the curriculum, the raising of the community's view of nursing education thus elevating standards, and the encouragement of nurses to return to school, all through the professional model which the master's-prepared faculty exhibited. Specific changes were noted such as development of new baccalaureate and associate degree nursing programs and the closure of hospital-based diploma programs in accord with the position taken by the nursing organizations. Alumnae in the first few programs noted the National League for Nursing accreditation received by some of the local schools of nursing, and the development of baccalaureate outreach programs within the region to assist nurses to achieve that degree if they had not obtained it as part of their basic education.

Comments from the graduates are noted in the following samples:

Nursing school is impacted by the quality of the faculty. Students see better role models. They get an expanded idea of what nursing can do and sense a greater ability to achieve these goals.

(Faculty) credentials are comparable to other faculty. Their increased creditability contributes to the total college.

In developing new educational programs, the community looked to us for leadership.

Nursing Service

There is general agreement that nursing service has improved through raising the level and quality of health services. More variability in response is noted in this question than occurred with the previous question which appeared to be related more to specific agency experiences than to a general reaction. Some agencies readily accepted the new graduates and changes resulted. In some agencies, master's preparation became a requirement for some of the positions. Sample comments are:

Agencies are hiring people with higher degrees—they're more willing to have nurses in expanded roles.

Presence of MSN helped nursing become more what it should be—patient-oriented, not task-oriented.

MSN graduates have found or created positions in health care agencies.

Nursing care services in the community have improved.

Graduates are involved in education, consultation, direct care, and research.

It's difficult to imagine what community would be like without these resourceful people.

The strongest support for changes in the delivery of nursing services was noted in the response of the graduates from the Western Michigan program. Some responders see changes in nursing service proceeding at a slower pace because pockets of resistance occur. Sample comments:

The impact is of lesser consequence. Some nurses have taken risks and established independent practice. Greater impact will occur later.

No dramatic change was noted.

Slow conservative community. Change will occur as we increase visibility and credibility in the community.

The local hospital doesn't allow the program to influence nursing care service.

There's some reluctance in some nursing administrators to accept MSN nurse.

Numerous comments are focused on the advent of the clinical nurse specialist in health care agencies. Respondents cite creative endeavors in practice undertaken by outreach graduates in their communities, including: development of nurse-run clinics, influence on a mental health agency and other services connected with courts and child protection, development of a screening program for scoliosis in the schools, promotion of family-centered maternity care in a local hospital, and consultation service to various agencies.

Image of Nursing in the Community

There is general agreement that the image of nursing in the community has been enhanced as a result of the demonstrated knowledge and expertise which the graduates exhibit in their relationships in the community with other health care providers and consumers. The advanced preparation is respected by colleagues in other disciplines although several respondents commented on the threat that the psychiatric and mental health nurses were to others who provide therapy such as social workers and counselors. Relationships with physicians vary and appear to be a function of a particular situation, with some based on a colleagueship role while others tend to be based on the role of the nurse as a handmaid or as a physician extender. In general, comments were favorable to the type of relationship which is developing.

Some respondents expressed frustration with the slowness of the change in image, but do note evidence of an evolving favorable image in their community. A few note no change in community relationships.

The nurse as a model of a competent professional is stated as the most significant factor in changing the image of nursing. Several note that the change that they have been able to effect has now raised the image of the baccalaureate nurse in their communities. Sample comments are:

> High school students were impressed that nursing is such a scholarly and legitimate profession.

> Image seems more and more as enhanced by roles graduates take. For the most part, they are accepted as competent, professional people on par with other health care providers.

> Public is slowly gaining more respect for added skills expertise of nurses providing care.

> Medical community beginning to see us more positively.

> Encountered resistance in agency from staff who saw nurse in a traditional role.

> Many of my clients relieved they have a nurse with advanced education.

> Changes are slow in our conservative community.

From the perspective of the alumnae, the most dramatic change in their communities since the outreach program left the area are related to nursing education. Practice changes are variable in accord with values in a region, but they result from the practice model portrayed by the graduates and the trickle down effect of the improvement in nursing education. The nursing image is being enhanced through the professional knowledge and expertise demonstrated by master's-prepared nurses, the faculty in schools of nursing, and the practitioners in various health care delivery systems.

Data reported suggest indeed the Master of Science Outreach Program offered by the College of Nursing in the four sites of Michigan have had a significant impact on the entire scope of nursing wherever the program was located. The major changes are a function of time, but all the changes reported have occurred in ten years or less. Of note is not only the actual changes that occurred, but also the energy and motivation which has been released so that continued changes through the efforts of the graduates and their colleagues will be a feature of the future.

Change is not only pronounced in areas of education and practice, but in the climate and value system which permeates the nursing community and thus influences the health care climate in the entire community. Even where changes have been few, the graduates express belief that changes will come about in time. The "mass inoculation" of a cohort of nurses prepared at the graduate level did make a difference, a significant qualitative indicator of the outreach endeavor.

An important dimension of a qualitative evaluation of an outreach program is the type of impact such an endeavor had on the sponsoring institution. The focus here is the impact on the people involved, the mission of the sponsoring institution, and the image of the institution in the larger community. An outreach endeavor calls on a tremendous investment of competence, energy, time, and commitment. In the instance of the College of Nursing and Wayne State University, the expenditures extended over a 12-year period.

Faculty

Faculty and other personnel directly involved in the effort gained stature in the state as their expertise and professional experiences were shared with a broader range of students. Many became a part of the network of the graduates as they were sought for consultation, presentation of research, and other papers at professional meetings in the regions and for professional advisement as the graduates moved through the various stages of their careers. Faculty also augmented their own knowledge base as they taught in a milieu different from their usual circumscribed environment on campus and in surrounding agencies. They explored new teaching strategies and took greater risks as they experienced multiple ways of achieving a goal. Recognition that one was now on the "students' turf" was also influenced by community values and practices providing a new perspective of the knowledges shared in the setting.

The program evaluators sought information at the close of each program as to faculty's perception of the significance of the experience. The first evaluation report at the conclusion of the first two outreach programs stated, "Faculty felt that the outreach programs are feasible, better than proliferating poor graduate programs, and essential (though not the only means) if nursing is to advance." This position was maintained in general by faculty in the other programs and their satisfaction, in addition to that associated with helping students learn and develop, was their contribution in helping to fill a need in the nursing community.

Sponsoring Institution

Both the College of Nursing and Wayne State University were influenced by this outreach endeavor. Wayne State University is an urban university, but historically, it has responded to requests to bring its resources to the larger community in the state. This nursing program however has been its most intensive, long-term effort throughout the state.

At the conclusion of the first program, the president and assistant provost of the university were interviewed relative to their perception of the outreach program. In citing the university's past efforts, and expressing a favorable position on outreach programs, they stated that decisions about such programs are viewed with care for two main reasons: they are visible programs which reflect on the university's reputation and because they generally require outside funding. The administration was very satisfied with the outreach program. They felt that standards had been upheld and the program benefited the community through the upgrading of nursing skills in the Upper Peninsula.

When the outreach program in the Upper Peninsula began, there was a statement in the 1975 Michigan Annual Operating Appropriation Act for Higher Education, Section 4, sub section a, which was of concern to institutions of higher learning where considerations were being given to offer outreach programs. The language of the statement is:

(4) Only on-campus enrollments shall be counted for funding purposes.

Funded on-campus enrollments shall be limited to the following:

(a) Student credit hours applicable toward a baccalaureate or graduate degree which are taught in facilities physically located within the boundaries of the campus as defined by the campus master plan as reviewed by the joint capital outlay subcommittee.

This matter was under discussion at the state level.

The director of the outreach program had the opportunity to meet the state representative for the Upper Peninsula region who also was the chairman of the senate appropriations committee, and drew his attention to this act and the implications it had for the nurses in that region and other areas of the state who could not access graduate programs in nursing which were located in the southeastern part of the state. On his suggestion, a letter relative to this matter was sent from the outreach director after consultation with the Wayne State University state government liaison officer to him and to the chairman of the House Appropriations Committee.

The statement was not continued in the 1976 appropriations bill. Student credit hours generated were permitted for funding, but not new degree programs not approved by the legislature. Although one cannot say that this instance is a result of cause and effect, certainly the implications of the act as it affected students in the outreach program were a factor in demonstrating its limitations.

The image of the college of nursing and the university has been enhanced through this outreach program. The program was cited in the Institute of Medicine Report (1983), *Nursing and Nursing Education: Public Policies and Private Actions:*

Examples (of outreach programs) include California State University at Fresno, Montana State University, and University of Maryland (offering baccalaureate degree training to RNs with associate degree and diploma) and Wayne State University (offering master's degree preparation to RNs in remote areas of Michigan). (p. 163)

The director was invited to deliver five major papers on outreach programming at national professional meetings.

Some Approaches to Master's Education in Nursing. Keynote address. American Association of Colleges of Nursing. March, 1980, Lexington, Kentucky.

Conserving Education Resources: A Community-Based Model for an Outreach Master's Program in Nursing. American Academy of Nursing. September, 1980, Dallas, Texas.

Community-Based Model for Outreach Programs. Nurse Educator Conference. November, 1980, San Francisco, California.

A Community-Based Model for Outreach Programs. First Annual Nursing Education Research Scientific Conference. January, 1983, San Francisco, California.

Impact of Outreach Master of Science in Nursing Program. Fifth Annual Scientific Conference of the Society for Research in Nursing Education. January, 1987, San Francisco, California.

The first two papers were published by the organization sponsoring the programs.

Other evidence of the reputation on the College of Nursing, Wayne State University, in the development of outreach programs is the invitation extended to the director to serve as a consultant to eight other universities which were providing for outreach programs. The continuous renewal of funding for the various programs by the Division of Nursing, Department of Health and Human Resources as it operated within its policies and guidelines evidenced the recognition of the quality and significance of the outreach program to nursing. The division also used the College of Nursing's model in assisting other programs as they explored the possibility of offering outreach programs.

The contribution the College of Nursing has made to nursing in Michigan is acknowledged and respected by many groups. The program prepared 257 nurses at the graduate level, many who would not have the opportunity to reach this achievement. (The fifth program was concluded in June, 1987 so the first graduates of that group received their degrees in May, 1987.) Throughout the state, the College of Nursing is recognized for its willingness to and perseverance in taking a risk to help so many communities improve the health services provided by their nurses. When the college celebrated its 40th anniversary in April, 1985, its outreach contribution to the state was cited in the Certificate of Special Tribute from the State of Michigan which was signed by the governor, James Blanchard. It reads:

> The college pioneered the Nursing Outreach Program which expands the opportunity for a Master's Degree in Nursing through the establishment of WSU centers throughout the State of Michigan. This program has been cited in a report to the United States Congress as a model for making graduate study more accessible to nurses in underserved areas.

In 1979, the Department of Education in Michigan conducted a study to make recommendations about nursing education at the graduate level. The Wayne State University outreach model was selected as the appropriate model to meet the needs of nurses removed from metropolitan areas in the state.

The success of the outreach endeavor in the first program was recognized by the Kellogg Foundation and the director of the outreach program received a grant to conduct a similar type of program for nurses from associate degree and diploma programs so that they could earn a baccalaureate degree in nursing. This program was designed for the Greater Detroit Metropolitan area and offered a setting away from the main campus close to where the nurses lived and worked.

Since the closure of the last outreach program, the College of Nursing has developed a metro outreach master's program which is offered in the far western part of the Detroit Metropolitan area. Using the same model with emphasis on weekend teaching, it is meeting the need of employed commuting nurses in and beyond the immediate western region.

The outreach program has impacted on the sponsoring college and university. Outreach teaching is an accepted means of reaching a population with limited access to the regularly scheduled programs on the main campus. Faculty enter this endeavor with commitment and full resolve to ensure that all programs so offered meet the standards reflective of the highest quality. The college and university are recognized as resources to those who wish to engage in outreach programming and their accountability is acknowledged by all who have been involved during the past 12 years. The programs were in accord with the mission of the university and enhanced its image on a regional, state, and international level.

RECOMMENDATIONS FOR PERSONS PLANNING GRADUATE PROFESSIONAL OUTREACH PROGRAMS

What lessons were learned from the experiences of the College of Nursing, Wayne State University, that would be helpful to individuals who plan outreach programs, especially those in professional fields which also have a practice component?

Faculty suggestions to administrators thinking of implementing a similar outreach program include:

Be prepared to be flexible.

Provide adequate planning before program starts.

Provide for good administrative support.

Guarantee quality by using on-campus faculty.

Export the total program.

Acquire community involvement.

The graduates were asked for two types of information: the actions of the College of Nursing which facilitated the attainment of their degree and the suggestions that they would make to someone contemplating such an endeavor.

There is a remarkable consistency among all groups in the ranking of actions taken by the College of Nursing which contributed toward attainment of their goal (see Table 27).

The ranking portrayed in the table represents actions receiving 50 percent or more responses from graduates. Stress is an inherent part of any graduate study, especially when persons who have been self-directed and responsible for decisions in work and life assume the dependent role of students. This change in life pattern becomes even more exaggerated in outreach programs where direct access to the "parent institution" is not available.

Actions which recognize the life demands on students and the responsible roles they play in their life eliminate much of the bureaucratic hassle and provide for a "caring about" atmosphere for their concerns. Programs which enable students to use resources of the community are also considered valuable in facilitating the outreach student's ability to handle the inherent stressors and complete the degree requirements.

Many of the suggestions graduates offered were elaborations on the actions which were the strengths of the program in meeting the goals of the students. Some general comments were expressed by the responders. Many feel that the community-based model which the College of Nursing developed and refined should be replicated by others. There was a plea that when people come into a community with the program they make a concerted effort to know who the students are and the roles they assume in their communities. This implies recognition of them as adult learners who have individual experiences to bring to the program in spite of the sometime geographic isolation where they live and work. One word, *flexibility*, was repeated throughout the responses, whether related to program and scheduling of courses and classes or in the admission criteria used. Because of other demands on their time and energy, it is most important that the students receive a total plan of courses at the start of the program.

Students mentioned the need for attention to the publicity about the program so that its accessibility is known by the appropriate population. With the notion of publicity is the provision for sufficient lead time for the start up of the program once it is announced. Time must be sufficient for student deficits to be addressed and their life plans adjusted to include the new activities involved. There was some criticism about the time needed between the announcement of the outreach program by the College of Nursing and the onset of courses (less than a full term). The short lead time resulted from the timing of the grant funding and the total time span available to complete a program in an outreach site (two or three years). Although plans could be in place and potential students notified of the possibility of the outreach program, no public announcements could be made until official

Table 27
Ranking of Facilitative Actions of the College of Nursing

Ranking	Total	UP	WM	HSA VI	HSA VII
1	Schedule	Schedule	Cognates courses in local universities	Schedule	Financial assistance
2	Cognate courses in local institutions	Faculty support	Schedule	Cognate courses in local institutions	Schedule
3	Faculty support	Cognate courses in local institutions	Faculty support	On-site registration	Cognate courses in local institutions
4	On-site registration	On-site registration	On-site registration	Faculty support	On-site registration
5	Financial assistance	Financial assistance	Access to library materials	Financial assistance	Faculty support
6	Access to library materials	Access to library materials	On-site office staff	Access to library materials	On-site office staff

word of funding was received. A prolonged delay from the awarding of the grant to the onset of classes could mean that the total program could not be completed. In such a situation, if the grant is essential to maintaining the program in the outreach site, then one needs to so notify the students as to what part will be guaranteed and measures developed to complete the programs. The short lead time for the College of Nursing outreach program did decrease the potential numbers of students. The short lead-time issue is related to granting procedures and is beyond remedy by the institution unless the sponsoring institution is willing to offer a promise.

Respondents also drew attention to the significance of the orientation program which is provided for the community. They suggested that the program and the demands it poses on the students and their families be discussed in an open, honest manner and that students recognize the commitment that such a program requires. This emphasis is particularly significant in graduate study. For example, some students were not prepared for the transition from undergraduate to graduate study. Students also need to be notified if the program is to be full time, part time, or a combination of both, and the meaning of these terms.

Other suggestions related to the practices used in the College of Nursing program: use of well-qualified on-campus faculty who are motivated to teach outreach students and who teach a similar course on campus; offering of the same course and program as on campus (no watering down of the program requirements); a strong on-site office with a coordinator willing to listen and a good system of communication; and a careful screening of on-site clinical faculty to be sure they can meet the same standards as other faculty. One other consideration which may arise in planning is the decision as to how many students should be accommodated in a program. The College of Nursing program decided to accept any eligible students who applied. This decision reflected two factors: the program would be in the area only once, thus it was important to reach as many students as possible; and a large part of the costs are fixed regardless of how many students were enrolled. The administrative staff, supplies, and communication systems are essential. The major alterable variables are the number of faculty and travel costs. The number of faculty most influenced by increase in size of student group are the clinical faculty who are responsible for the supervision of students. Their costs are not remarkable since they are part time and do not require the more costly fringe benefits. Travel has to be recognized as an increase, but often faculty travel to the area together and costs are shared. The pay-off in using the outreach structure for large numbers of students is really a cost-effective process.

CONCLUSION

A graduate program in a professional health field has a unique opportunity to be a catalyst for change in outreach sites often far removed from university medical centers. By teaching the students within their own communities, they become the change agents and introduce new ideas and practices in concert with the values and mores of the community. This mechanism avoids a perceived "imperialistic" approach which may occur when outsiders come into a community with the intent of imposing their "new" ideas on a community.

Communities where the outreach programs are located and where the graduates are practicing are undergoing changes in health and nursing care and its delivery to its citizens. Most changes are the result of changing health care economics, but others are the result of the professional model the graduates exhibit through their knowledge and expertise. The greatest change occurred in the educational area where schools of nursing with prepared faculty are now nationally accredited and the communities have more professional nursing programs in their colleges and universities. Changes in practice are also underway through the efforts of the graduates and through the practice of the new graduates from the now accredited nursing schools in the community.

The College of Nursing and Wayne State University have also been changed as a result of their risk-taking and perseverance in bringing the outreach graduate program to a nursing population outside the immediate range of graduate programs in nursing in the state. The College of Nursing has received recognition and high praise from the nursing community in the state and nationally and is acknowledged to be an important resource to others who seek to embark on such an endeavor. Cited in official documents and reported at national meetings and in the nursing literature, the outreach program has made a significant contribution to nursing and nursing education.

The community-based model for the outreach program which was developed and refined by the College of Nursing was a most effective framework and has been recommended for replication by other institutions. The model guided the decision making so that responsibilities for various components of the program were clearly delineated, the community involvement prevented duplication and kept costs within a reasonable limit, and the programs presented were directed toward the needs of a particular student body while maintaining the integrity and quality of the graduate program.

The Master of Science in Nursing Outreach Program provided by the College of Nursing, Wayne State University, did have an impact on all who were involved and has demonstrated that a quality graduate professional educational program can be offered in an outreach model.

References*

Argyris, C., & Shon, D. (1974). *Theory and practice: Increasing professional effectiveness.* San Francisco: Jossey-Bass.

Bowen, H. (1973). Financing the external degree. *Journal of Higher Education, 44,* 479–493.

Brinkman, P. T. (1981). Factors affecting instructional costs of major research universities. *Journal of Higher Education, 52,* 265–276.

Broderius, B., & Carder, M. (1983). Delivering a non-resident master's degree: Qualitative and quantitative measures of effectiveness. *Alternative Higher Education, 7,* 116–132.

Brown, R. D., & Krager, L. (1985). Ethical issues in graduate education: Faculty and student responsibility. *Journal of Higher Education, 56,* 403–418.

Brown, E., & Lyons, J. M. (1982). *Analyzing the cost of baccalaureate nursing education.* New York: National League for Nursing.

Carnegie Commission of Higher Education (1971). *Higher education and the nation's health.* New York: McGraw-Hill.

Conrad, C., & Pratt, A. (1985). Designing for quality. *Journal of Higher Education, 56,* 601–622.

Council on Postsecondary Accreditation (1983). *Policy statement on off-campus credit programs.* Washington, DC: Council on Post Secondary Accreditation.

---

* These reference citations include those used both in text and those significant to the topic of concern.

Cross, K. (1973). The external degree: Introduction. *Journal of Higher Education, 44,* 415–425.

Cross, K. (1981). *Adults as learners.* San Francisco: Jossey-Bass.

Diers, D. (1985). Preparation of practitioners, clinical specialists and clinicians. *Journal of Professional Nursing, 1,* 41–47.

Dressel, P. (1979). External and non-traditional graduate programs. *Peabody Journal of Education, 56,* 210–211.

Eisley, J. C., & Coppard, L. C. (1977). *Feasibility study of external graduate degree programs: Extending opportunities for graduate studies in Michigan.* Ann Arbor, MI: Horace H. Rackham School of Graduate Studies, University of Michigan.

Forni, P., & Walsh, M., (1987). The professional versus the academic model: A dilemma for nursing education. *Journal of Professional Nursing, 5,* 291–297.

Grossman, D. M. (1987). Electronic college courses: The professor must be in charge. *The Chronicle of Higher Education, 33,* 22, 104.

Gunne, C. (1985). Fiscal status of nursing education programs in U. S. *Journal of Professional Nursing, 1,* 336–347.

Harten, C., & Boyer, R. (1985). Administrator's receptive to non-traditional goals. *Journal of Higher Education, 56,* 206–219.

Halonen, R. J., Fitzgerald, J., & Simmon, K. (1978). Measuring the cost of clinical education. *Journal of Allied Health, 7,* 192–198.

Institute of Medicine (1977). *Costs of education in health professions.* Washington, DC: National Academy of Medicine.

Institute of Medicine, Committee on Nursing and Nursing Education (1983). *Nursing and nursing education: Public policies and private actions.* Washington, DC: National Academy Press.

Johnson, L. (1978). *Receptivity and resistance. Faculty response to the external degree at the University of Michigan.* Unpublished doctoral dissertation, University of Michigan, Ann Arbor.

Kelley, J., & Flowers, J. (1985). An innovative approach to graduate education in nursing. *Journal of Professional Nursing, 1,* 238–243.

Klippick, A. L. et al. (1978). *Evaluation of a baccalaureate external degree program in health service administration with major in long term care administration* (BBBI0787) Bethesda, MD. Division of Associated Health Professions, Health Resources Administration (DHEW/PHS).

Knowles, M. et al. (1984). *Andrology in action: Applying modern principles of adult learning.* San Francisco: Jossey-Bass.

Kummer, K., Bednash, G., & Redman, B. (1987). Cost model for baccalaureate education. *Journal of Professional Nursing, 3,* 176–187.

Kuramato, A. (1978). The status of non-traditional study. *Journal of Continuing Education in Nursing, 9,* 29–32.

Lefferts, G. (1977). Alternative to higher education. *CEPF Journal, 15,* 8–9, 18.

Lenburg, C. (1984). An update on the regents external degree program. *Nursing Outlook, 32,* 250–254.

McArt, E. (1987). Research facilitation in academic and practice settings. *Journal of Professional Nursing, 3,* 84–96.

McClothin, W. (1960). *Patterns of professional education.* New York: G. P. Putnam.

McGill, C., & Molinaro, L. (1978). Setting up and operating outreach centers for continuing education in nursing. *Journal of Continuing Education in Nursing, 9,* 14–18.

McKevitt, R. (1986). Trends in master's education in nursing. *Journal of Professional Nursing, 2,* 225–233.

Nolan, D. J. (1977). Open assessment in higher education: The New York regents external degree. *International Review of Education, 23,* 231–248.

Nursing, a social policy statement. (1980). Kansas City, MO: American Nurses' Association.

Reilly, D. E. (1980). *One approach to master's education in nursing.* Washington, DC: American Academy of Nursing.

Reilly, D. E. (1981). Conserving educational resources: A community-based model for an outreach master's program in nursing. In American Academy of Nursing, *Impact of Changing Resources Health Policy* (pp. 49–64). Kansas City, MO: American Academy of Nursing.

Reilly, D. E. (1985). *The clinical field: Its use in nursing education.* Norwalk, CT: Appleton-Century-Crofts.

Schein, E. H. (1972). *Professional education: Some new directions.* New York: McGraw-Hill.

Schlotfeldt, R. (1987). Reflection on nursing, 1987. *Nursing Outlook, 35,* 226–228.

Silverman, J. (1973). The external degree. *Journal of Higher Education, 56.*

Stark, J., Lowther, M., Hagerty, B., & Orezyk, C. (1986). A conceptual framework for the study of preservice professional programs in colleges and universities. *Journal of Higher Education, 56,* 601–622.

Strauss, M. (1979). *University without walls: External degree program. Final report* (bbb 12752) Bethesda, MD: Health Resources Administration, Bureau of Health Manpower.

Tennessee Higher Education Commission (1969). *Cost of collegiate education in Tennessee.* Nashville, TN: Tennessee Higher Education Commission.

Todd, F. (1982). *Budgeting.* Unpublished course syllabus.

Warren, J. (1973). External degrees: Coping with the problems of credit. *Journal of Higher Education, 44,* 465–478.

Whitten, B. K. (1978). Teaching graduate physiology in a remote area. *The Physiologist, 21* (6).

Appendix A

Questionnaire for Alumnae Master of Science in Nursing Outreach Program

College of Nursing
Wayne State University

PART I

I DEMOGRAPHIC INFORMATION

Name _____
       (while in program)

Address _____

         _____

         _____.

Is address same as when you were in the program? Yes ____ No ____
If no, please indicate

    Street, etc. _____

    City, State _____

Have you moved from Michigan since completing your program?
    Yes ____ No ____
If yes, please complete the following:

Location   **Dates**

_____   _____

_____   _____

177

_____   _____

_____   _____

Age when you started program _____

Family status while in the program (Circle appropriate one)
1 Single
2 Married
3 Widowed
4 Divorced
5 Separated

Children: Number _____ Age Range _____

Undergraduate degree at time of entry (Circle appropriate one and complete)

Type	Graduation Date
1 BSN/BS(N) Accredited by NLN	_____
2 BSN/BS(N) Unaccredited by NLN	_____
3 Other (Specify)	_____

II PROGRAM

(Circle appropriate one and complete)

	Completion Date	Projected Completion Date
1 Upper Peninsula 1975–77	_____	_____
2 Western Michigan 1977–80	_____	_____
3 HSA VI (Tri City) 1980–82	_____	_____
4 HSA VII (N.West. Michigan) 1982–85	_____	_____

MAJOR   (Circle appropriate one)
1 Community Health Nursing
2 Advanced Medical-Surgical Nursing
3 Advanced Maternity Nursing
4 Health Care of Women
5 Adult-Psychiatric-Mental Health Nursing
6 Teaching

MINOR   (Circle appropriate one)

1   Teaching
2   Administration
3   Clinical (Specify)
4   None

III EMPLOYMENT

	Title	Full-Time Part-Time	Agency	Dates
A. Entry into program	_____	_____	_____	_____
Present	_____	_____	_____	_____

B. Positions held since the completion of the Master's Program (please put latest one first). If you have not completed the program, use the official termination date of the program in your area.

Position Title	Full-Time Part-Time	Agency	Dates From–To
_____	_____	_____	_____
_____	_____	_____	_____
_____	_____	_____	_____
_____	_____	_____	_____
_____	_____	_____	_____

C. Reasons for change to the latest position (Circle appropriate one)

1   Advancement
2   Greater opportunity
3   Need for new experience
4   Dissatisfaction with previous experience
5   Spouse's relocation to different area
6   Increased salary
7   More compatible with my preparation
8   Personal
9   Other (Specify) _____

D. The earning of my master's degree influenced the change(s) in my positions (Circle the appropriate one)

1   Significantly
2   Somewhat
3   Not at all

If answer is #1 or #2, answer below

Changes were in (Circle the appropriate one(s) and rank in importance)

Rank

    1 Pay increase

    2 Recognition

    3 Role

    4 Choice in options

    5 Other (Specify) _____

If answer is #3, clarify _____

E. Is your present position congruent with your goal in nursing?

Yes _____ No _____ Partially _____

If not yes, please describe the ideal position for you _____

_____

_____

_____

What factors are deterring you from seeking that position? (Circle the appropriate one(s))

    1 Lack of mobility

    2 Limited opportunity in the area

    3 More advanced study required

    4 Lack of needed funds for further study

    5 Lack of educational resources in the area

    6 Lack of motivation

    7 Personal

    8 Other

F. Has your degree influenced the income you now receive from working?

Yes _____ No _____

If yes, what was the increase? (Circle correct amount)

    1 0–$999

    2 $1,000–$4,999 per year

    3 $5,000–$9,999 per year

    4 $10,000–$15,000 per year

    5 Over $15,000

If no, what is the reason? (Circle correct one(s))

1 Set pay scale in area
2 No recognition
3 No change in job
4 Other (Specify) _____

IV   ADVANCED STUDY

A. Have you been or are you currently enrolled in a doctorate program?

Yes _____ No _____

If yes, circle the appropriate one and complete

Degree	Institution	Entry Date	Completion Date	Projected Completion Date
1 PhD in nursing	_____	_____	_____	_____
2 D.Nursing Science	_____	_____	_____	_____
3 PhD (Specify)	_____	_____	_____	_____
4 EdD	_____	_____	_____	_____
5 Other (Specify)	_____	_____	_____	_____

If you have not enrolled in a doctoral program, do you plan to do so?

Yes _____ No _____

If yes, what degree will you be pursuing? (Circle appropriate one and complete)

Type of Degree	Institution	Projected Starting Date
1 PhD in nursing	_____	_____
2 D.Nursing Science	_____	_____
3 PhD (Specify)	_____	_____
4 EdD	_____	_____

5   Other (Specify) _____   _____

Why will you be pursuing this advanced study? (Circle the two major reasons)

1   Advancement in position
2   New opportunities
3   Continued intellectual and professional stimulation
4   Economic advantages
5   Other (Specify) _____

B. Certificate Programs

Have you earned a post master's certificate?   Yes ____ No ____

If yes, circle the appropriate one(s) and complete

		Place	Date
1	Administration	_____	____
2	Gerontology	_____	____
3	Critical Care Nursing	_____	____
4	Midwifery	_____	____
5	Pediatric	_____	____
6	Neonatal Nursing	_____	____
7	Oncology/Oncology Nursing	_____	____
8	Other (Specify)	_____	____

C. Seminars, Professional Meetings Attended for Continuing Education

Topic	Sponsor	Date
_____	_____	____
_____	_____	____
_____	_____	____
_____	_____	____
_____	_____	____

D. Certification

Have you taken tests for certification?   Yes ____ No ____

Are you currently certified?   Yes ____ No ____

If yes, circle appropriate one(s) and complete

Area	**Sponsor**	**Date**
1 Medical Surgical Nursing	_____	_____
2 Psychiatric/Mental Health Nursing	_____	_____
3 Pediatric Nursing	_____	_____
4 Occupational Health Nursing	_____	_____
5 Critical Care Nursing	_____	_____
6 Maternity Nursing	_____	_____
7 Nursing Administration	_____	_____
8 Other	_____	_____

V PUBLICATIONS

Have you published since completing program? Yes _____ No _____

If yes, please circle appropriate one(s) and complete

	Title and Publisher	**Date**
1 Book	_____	_____
2 Chapter(s) of a book	_____	_____
3 Editor of Book	_____	_____
4 Monograph	_____	_____
5 Abstract	_____	_____
6 Journal refereed	_____	_____
	_____	_____
	_____	_____
7 Journal non-refereed	_____	_____
	_____	_____
	_____	_____

VI RESEARCH

Have you participated in any research since completion of the program?

Yes _____ No _____ If yes, please complete the following:

Topic	Sponsor	Date

Funding of research (Circle appropriate one(s))

1   Division of Nursing—USPHS
2   Employing institution
3   Health organization (Specify) _____
4   Community group (Specify) _____
5   Other (Specify) _____
6   None

VII   PRESENTATIONS AT PROFESSIONAL MEETINGS

Have you made any presentations at professional meetings (local, state, national) since you entered the master's program?

Yes _____ No _____

If yes, complete the following—list in chronological order

Topic and Sponsor	Date	Invited, or Refereed, or Solicited

VIII   HONORS

Have you been the recipient of any honors since you entered the masters' program? Yes _____ No _____

If yes, what is the source and title? Circle the appropriate one and complete

1   Sigma Theta Tau _____
2   State Nurses Association _____
3   National Nurses Association _____
4   Local Nurses Association _____

    5 University/School/Health Agency _____

    6 Community _____

    7 Other _____

IX MEMBERSHIP INTO PROFESSIONAL ORGANIZATIONS

Do you currently have membership in a professional organization?

Yes _____ No _____

If yes, circle the appropriate one(s)

    1 American Nurses' Association
    2 National League for Nursing
    3 American Public Health Association
    4 Critical Care Nursing Association
    5 Operating Room Nurses Association
    6 Occupational Health Nurses Association
    7 Sigma Theta Tau
    8 Other (Specify) _____

In which of the above organizations did you hold membership *before* *entering* the master's program?

_____

_____

_____

_____

Which of the above organizations have you joined since entering the master's program?

_____

_____

_____

_____

Have you held positions of responsibility in any of these organizations? Yes _____ No _____

If yes, what position? (Circle correct response(s) and answer)

		Since entering the program? Yes	No
1	President	—	—
2	Other Officer	—	—
3	Task Force Member	—	—

4   Program Planning Member   __ __

5   Committee Member (Specify) _____   __ __

6   Other (Specify) _____   __ __

Since graduation from the program, have you attended any Michigan Nurses Association Conventions, either fully or partially?

Yes ____ No ____

If yes, circle the appropriate number

1   1 convention
2   2–3 conventions
3   4 or more conventions

X   COMMUNITY ACTIVITY

Have you been involved in health-related community activities since graduation from the program? Yes ____ No ____

If yes, what type of activity? (Circle appropriate one(s))

1   Teaching health matters to lay groups
2   Membership on boards
3   Leading group sessions
4   Teaching specialized groups (i.e., ENT)
5   Contributing articles to media
6   Other _____

XI   PROGRAM SIGNIFICANCE

How did the presence of the Outreach MSN program influence your decision to earn an MSN degree? (Circle appropriate one(s))

1   I would have the degree anyway
2   I would eventually earn the degree
3   I would not be able to obtain the degree
4   I would have earned a master's degree outside nursing
5   Other (Specify) _____

In what ways did the College of Nursing facilitate your attainment of the master of science degree in nursing? Circle the appropriate one(s) below

1   Class schedule to accommodate work patterns
2   Accessibility of library materials in the region
3   Faculty support

4   Financial assistance
5   Accessibility of an on-site office and staff
6   Communication system
7   On-site registration procedure
8   Acceptance of cognate and elective courses from local
    universities
9   Other _____

What words of advice would you offer to a school planning to initiate
an Outreach program?

Comments:

PART II
IMPACT OF THE PROGRAM

The following two questions seek to address the question: What is the
"pay-off" of an intensive educational university program to nurses in the
community? The viewpoints of those most intimately involved in the experiences and the process of learning are valuable sources of data. Your willingness to respond to the questions below from *your perspective* will help us to
understand the benefits or impact of the program. One question relates to you
and the other relates to the community. If you have left the community shortly
after finishing the program, you may or may not want to answer the questions
on the impact of the community.

Please respond to each question as fully and candidly as possible. Use
both sides of paper and feel free to use additional sheets of paper. While each
question suggests areas for you to consider, do not hesitate to add other
information if you choose. Indicate the nature of direction of the changes and
feel free to give some examples related to each question.

1.   To what extent has the program in which you participated changed
     — your professional goals, expectations?
     — your image of your self?
     — your relationship to the health care concerns of the community?

— your ability to see new or different insights and to grow?
— your viewpoints of nursing?
— your life in general?

2. To what extent has the program in which you participated
   — influenced nursing education in the community?
   — influenced the nursing care services in the community?
   — changed the image of nursing in the community or in the agencies
     which provide health care?

Appendix B
Clinical Course Evaluation Survey

Course
Number: _____ Quarter: _____ Year: _____ Instructor: _____

DIRECTIONS: Please fill in the spaces at the top of this form. Please circle the number of the response option of your choice. Leave blank if not applicable.

1. How was the setting for the clinical experience selected?
   (1) Basically, it was selected by me.
   (2) I jointly selected it with the instructor.
   (3) Basically, it was assigned to me by the instructor.

2. Rate the extent to which you were satisfied with the way your setting was selected.
   Very Dissatisfied 1 2 3 4 5 Very Satisfied

3. Estimate the number of *individual* conferences (face-to-face or by telephone) which you have had with your clinical course faculty.
   (1) Usually less than once per month.
   (2) Usually once per month.
   (3) Usually twice per month.
   (4) Usually once per week.
   (5) Usually more than once per week.

4. The average length of *individual* conferences was about _____ minutes.

5. Estimate the number of *group* sessions you had with your clinical faculty.
   (1) Usually less than once per month.
   (2) Usually once per month.
   (3) Usually twice per month.

(4)   Usually once per week.

(5)   Usually more than once per week.

6.   The average length of *group* conferences was about _____ minutes.

7.   Approximately how many times did your clinical faculty observe you in the clinical setting during this quarter? _____

8.   Please estimate the amount of time you spent (minutes or hours) on this clinical course per week excluding regularly scheduled class sessions:

_____ in the field setting

_____ reading or writing assignments

_____ other activities

Regarding Objectives for the Clinical Component of this Course:

9.   Objectives were:

Vague   1   2   3   4   5   Very clear

10.   Objectives were:

Not related to the   1   2   3   4   5   Strongly related to the
theory component   theory component

Regarding Clinical Instructional Assignments or Course Requirements:

11.   How valuable were course assigned readings for the clinical experience?

Useless   1   2   3   4   5   Very helpful

12.   Clinical instructional assignments in general were:

Poor learning   1   2   3   4   5   Very good learning
experiences   experiences

13.   Accessibility of instructional materials was:

Poor   1   2   3   4   5   Very good

Regarding Your Clinical Faculty for the Clinical Component of this Course:

14.   What was the feeling between the clinical faculty and the students?

Little mutual   1   2   3   4   5   Excellent mutual
understanding   understanding

15.   The clinical faculty's ability to make students feel free to ask questions or ask for help was:

Poor   1   2   3   4   5   Very good

16.   Concerning the clinical faculty's knowledge of the area, the faculty appeared to be:

Poorly informed   1   2   3   4   5   Extremely well informed

17. The clinical faculty's ability to answer student questions was

     Poor   1   2   3   4   5   Very good

18. The clinical faculty's knowledge of the agency(ies) setting and/or types of clients you worked with in this clinical course was:

     Poor   1   2   3   4   5   Very good

19. How well did the clinical faculty maximize the use of the agency or setting of the learning experience?

     Poor   1   2   3   4   5   Very well

20. The clinical faculty's demonstration of respect for students' skills, knowledge, and level of professional development was:

     Low   1   2   3   4   5   Very high

Regarding Supervision and Instructional Methods:

21. Clinical group conferences

     Useless   1   2   3   4   5   Very useful

22. How do you feel about the clinical faculty's supervisory methods?

     Dissatisfied   1   2   3   4   5   Very satisfied

23. How do you feel about the clinical faculty's instructional methods?

     Dissatisfied   1   2   3   4   5   Very satisfied

24. Individual conferences with the clinical faculty were:

     Useless   1   2   3   4   5   Very helpful

25. The availability of the clinical faculty for assistance was:

     Low   1   2   3   4   5   Very good

26. The work setting(s) in which conferences took place with clinical faculty were:

     Poor   1   2   3   4   5   Excellent

Regarding Student Evaluation and Feedback Procedures:

27. The criteria for evaluating your instructional assignments were:

     Vague   1   2   3   4   5   Exceptionally clear

28. Grading procedures for the course grade were:

     Unfair   1   2   3   4   5   Very fair

29. Feedback from the clinical faculty was such that:

     I never knew where I stood   1   2   3   4   5   I always knew where I stood

30. Verbal and/or written feedback from the clinical faculty regarding student's strengths and weaknesses was:

    Poor 1 2 3 4 5 Very good

31. The amount of time the faculty took to provide feedback of work turned in was:

    Too long 1 2 3 4 5 Very reasonable

In General:

32. Peer relationships among students in the course were:

    Poor 1 2 3 4 5 Very congenial

33. In relationship to the course objectives, the setting(s) of my clinical learning experience was:

    Inappropriate 1 2 3 4 5 Very appropriate

34. Overall, the clinical experience was:

    Poor 1 2 3 4 5 Excellent

35. Assess the overall effect of the clinical component of this course on your attitudes toward your program of study:

    Negative 1 2 3 4 5 Strongly positive

36. Specifically, what things in the clinical course would you suggest as being in need of change?

    _____

    _____

    _____

37. Specifically, what things in the clinical course do you feel should be kept as they are?

    _____

    _____

    _____

What general comments would you like to make about the clinical course experience?

    _____

    _____

    _____

    _____

Appendix C
Research Skills Questionnaire

The purpose of this survey is to secure your judgment of your level of competence in utilizing research skills in your profession. The results will be used to compare student ratings of their competence with research skills between outreach programs and on-campus programs. You will not be identified personally in any way.

DIRECTIONS: Please answer *all* questions, even if your research sequence did not inclu.. the material covered in the question. Circle the number of the response option of your choice.

1. In which program were you enrolled:

    (1) Upper Peninsula Outreach Program

    (2) Western Michigan Outreach Program

    (3) On-campus Program

2. Indicate all courses in which you were enrolled.

    (1) NUR 0795-Field Study

    (2) NUR 0796-Research Practicum

    (3) NUR 0899-Master's Thesis Research

3. Do you feel prepared to develop a researchable question to utilize research in seeking a solution to some professional problem?

    Ill prepared 1 2 3 4 5 Very prepared

4. Are you comfortable with your knowledge of how to make a literature search to discover what other people know about your professional problem?

    No knowledge 1 2 3 4 5 Very knowledgeable

5. Do you know where to look in efforts to find already existing data collection instruments?

    No knowledge 1 2 3 4 5 Very knowledgeable

6. What level of skill do you feel that you have to write an instrument to collect data?

    No skill   1   2   3   4   5   Very skillful

7. How prepared do you feel that you are to draw a proper sample of subjects (assuming that subjects are available)?

    Ill prepared   1   2   3   4   5   Very prepared

8. How prepared do you feel that you are to complete the statistical analysis of a typical data collection effort?

    Ill prepared   1   2   3   4   5   Very prepared

9. Do you feel capable of writing a quality summary report of the research, including display of tables of data results if applicable?

    Not capable   1   2   3   4   5   Very capable

10. How likely is it that you would engage in a literature search to discover what is known about a professional problem or procedure prior to your enacting steps to address the professional problem?

    Not likely   1   2   3   4   5   Very likely

11. How likely is it that you would engage in a research study to discover a solution to a professional problem or procedural concern?

    Not likely   1   2   3   4   5   Very likely